HANDL
MENO

C000174455

Finally, a doctor answers women's questions.

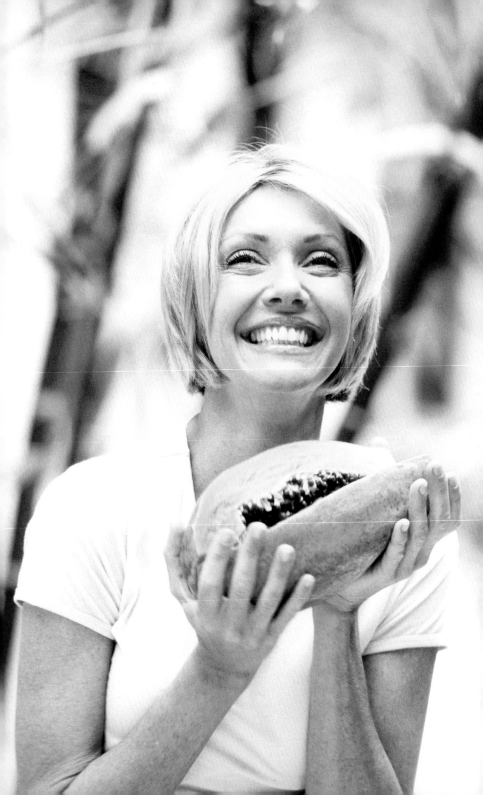

HANDLE YOUR MENOPAUSE

Finally, a doctor answers women's questions.

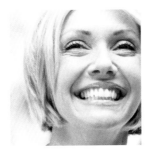

Dr Michèle Serrand

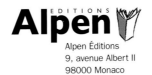

Alpen Éditions
9, avenue Albert II
98000 Monaco

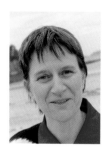

Michèle Serrand is a medical doctor and writer. She has practiced homeopathy for fifteen years. As president of Homéopathes Sans Frontières, she has taught the discipline to doctors and pharmacists in Africa and Asia.

Exclusive copyrights:
© Alpen Éditions
9, avenue Albert II
MC - 98000 MONACO
Tel: 00377 97 77 62 10
Fax: 00377 97 77 62 11
Web: www.alpen.mc

Managing Publisher: Christophe Didierlaurent
Editorial: Fabienne Desmarets and Sandra Del Barba
Designer: Stéphane Falaschi

Copyrights:
Eye Wire, Good Shoot, Photo Alto, Photo Disc, Digital Vision,
Image Source, Copyright © 20 N. Abdallah et
ses concédants : tous droits réservés

ISBN13: 978-2-35934-066-2

Printed in Italy

Introduction

In the Western world women most often approach menopause with anxiety. Women's magazines are full of the difficulties of this stage of life, and they stir up fears like the boogey man. These articles almost systematically conclude that all of menopause's difficulties will disappear by taking the hormone replacement therapy (HRT) proposed by the majority of gynecologists and general practitioners.

However, only 10 to 15% of women take HRT. Quite often, they stop it after the first year. This is for two reasons. First, they get tired of regularly ingesting chemicals. In addition, they fear the cancers linked to HRT, particularly breast cancer. Even though the pharmaceutical companies' words, relayed to women by the great majority of doctors, are reassuring, these women are cautious. Doctors tell us that the risk is minimal and that women treated with HRT receive better medical follow-up, which in turn promotes the early detection and treatment of tumours, leading to better prognoses. Despite all of these good arguments, women are wary. Arguments fluctuate, and the next thing you know, everyone is talking about the harmful effects of menopause, such as osteoporosis and heart disease, for example. Some claim that using HRT could prevent these harmful effects.

But what is menopause exactly? And what should we do about it? Are we condemned to choosing between the risk of breast cancer and the risk of fracturing a hipbone or femur or angina pectoris?

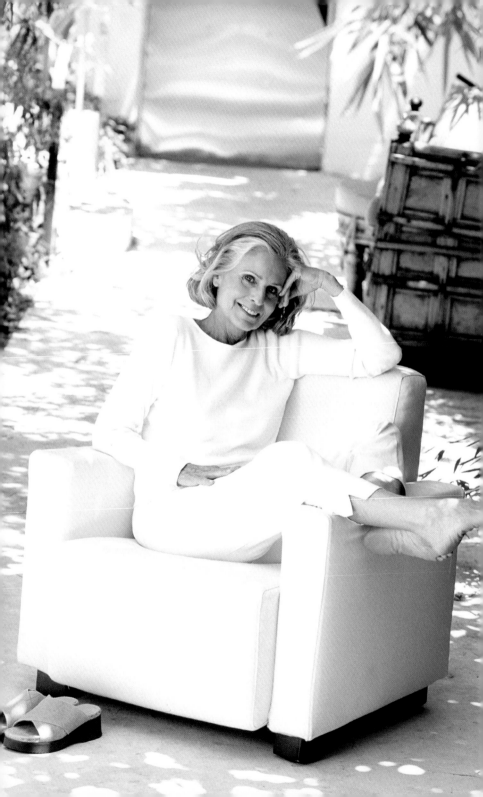

Is there a better way?

Do we perhaps have something to learn from Asian countries, particularly Japan?

Japanese women rarely suffer from hot fla s h e s. They have much less osteoporosis than Western women do. Researchers have shown that this advantage is linked to their diet, notably the presence of soy at every meal.

This book proposes to examine all of these questions in detail:

--First, what really is menopause?

--What are the advantages and disadvantages of chemical treatments: hormone replacement therapy, but also new treatments using SERMs (Selective Estrogen Receptor Modulators) and SASs (Selective Action Steroids)?

-- How can you feel at ease with yourself for choosing natural products to attain a new equilibrium in menopause?

Menopause can be a wonderful stage in women's lives. A certain art of living, which brings together a tasty diet, the rediscovery of movement, the practice of relaxation techniques, and the careful use of new functional foods rich in phytoestrogens like soy, helps women reach their peak.

CONTENTS

MENOPAUSE WITHOUT HRT : IS IT POSSIBLE?

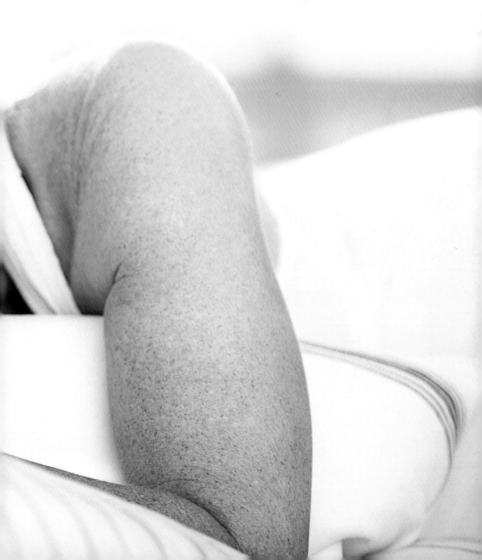

Menopause without HRT: is it possible?

For several months now, Martine has not been feeling well. "*It's menopause,*" says her best friend, Lydia, who has already been through it all.

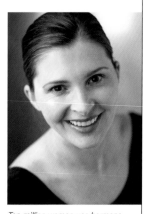

Ten million women use hormone replacement therapy. However, only 8% continue using it for more than two years.

Martine is irritable. Her nights have become unbearable. She wakes up several times through the night covered in sweat. So she undresses, but then starts to shiver. In the end, she pulls the comforter back on, falls back to sleep, and it all starts over again.

During the day, it is hardly any better. She is a teacher, and in the middle of her classes, she feels her cheeks turning red. A sensation of heat invades her. Then she starts to perspire. So she takes off her jacket and opens the window. Ten minutes later, she closes it again. Martine knows for sure what is happening to her. For the last four months, she has not had a period. "*It's menopause,*" explains her friend Lydia, who has already gone through it.

A new way to eat

How do you go about it? For health reasons, Martine cannot use the HRT that several of her friends have mentioned. Suddenly, she is scared because they have promised her a whole load of hardships: dry skin, decreased libido, brittle bones. All of this continually worries her and only increases her anxiety. Suddenly, at home, she is on edge, and things are getting more and more difficult with her partner..

"I can't use it either," says Lydia, *"and, look, I'm doing great. And I don't take any chemical medication. My doctor suggested a new way of eating. He urged me to change my lifestyle a bit, to do more sports, to take up relaxing activities. And he suggested soy-based dietary supplements. Since then, I've been doing very well. I don't have hot flashes anymore. I sleep better. During the day, I'm not irritable anymore. And I want to do lots of things."*

Yes, but for the heart and bones, is it enough?

"My doctor carefully explained that, by combining this diet with activity and by taking nutritional supplements, I'm also reducing the risks of having problems with my heart and bones. He pointed out some very good websites where it's all explained and where you can find the latest studies on these issues."

Martine regains her confidence. She is going to gather information and make an appointment with her doctor to take stock of the situation.

Prepare yourself for your appointment with the doctor

Your doctor has a great deal of knowledge about menopause and the treatments for it, but she or he cannot answer questions that you do not ask. That is why it is so important to prepare your conversation by taking the advice of friends who have already gone through menopause and those currently being treated. Gather as much information as possible from books, magazine articles, and certainly the internet, if you have access to it. Take a keen interest in the nutritional aspects of menopause and in phytotherapy, topics that generally are not discussed in a traditional medical consultation. This book will help you prepare the essential questions you need to ask.

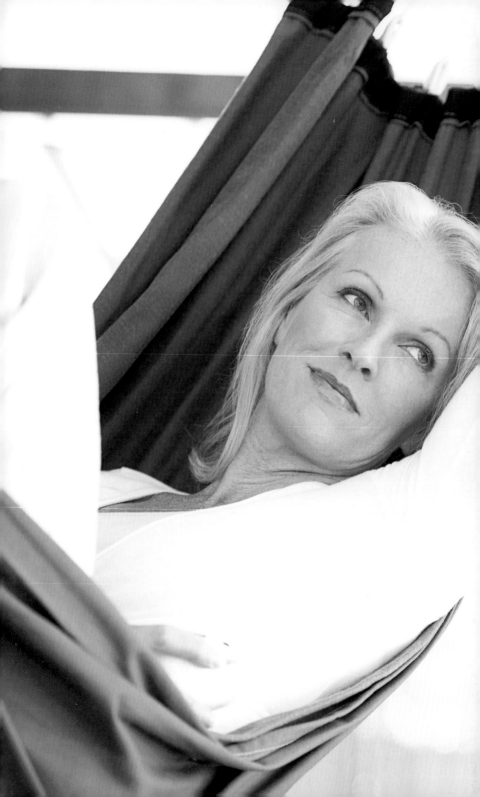

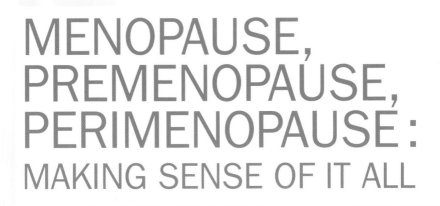

MENOPAUSE, PREMENOPAUSE, PERIMENOPAUSE:
MAKING SENSE OF IT ALL

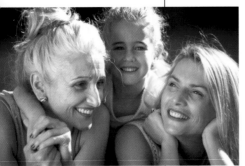

Understanding Women

In the female body, mobility, change, and adaptation are everything. Throughout every cycle, hormonal fluctuations and interactions give new meaning to the word "balance".

Menopause is the period in women's lives where menstruation stops. For many women, it brings a relief that is synonymous with freedom. However, for others, it is a sign of the advancing ye a r s, the approach of old age. Numerous fears are associated with it, notably, that of aging and no longer being seductive. Recognized for her wisdom in certain civilizations, the menopausal woman has to, from this point in her life onward, face the storm of hormonal imbalance that blows in during premenopause.

To understand better the phenomena of pre-menopause and menopause, it is best to return to the biological workings of menstruation. At birth, a female child has a certain number of dormant cells called oocytes in her ovaries.

The ovaries produce ova, which are destined for fertilization by sperm.

A cyclical phenomenon

At puberty, led by the action of hormones manufactured by the pituitary gland, a cyclical pattern begins, and every

28 days, on average, menstruation occurs. Menstrual periods occur when the mucosa of the uterus is shed when fertilization is absent. The first day of menstruation is the first day of the cycle. Each cycle consists of two parts: the first part, or follicular phase, which sees the development of a follicle in the ovary. This follicle secretes estrogens and contains an oocyte that will eventually become an ovum. Ovulation then follows; at this point, the follicle reaches maturity and bursts, thus releasing the ovum.

What follows in the second part of the cycle or the luteinic phase where progesterone is secreted promoting the development of uterine mucosa, whose purpose is to create a nest for an eventual egg. The egg is an ovum that has been fertilized by a spermatozoid.

In the absence of fertilization, the hormone levels of progesterone and estrogens drop, and the uterine mucus is shed, thereby creating a menstrual period.

This cyclical phenomenon is controlled by the pituitary gland, which is in turn controlled by the hypothalamus, which also responds to the blood levels of the two types of hormones manufactured by the ovaries: estrogens and progesterone. This entire process is very sensitive to neurotransmitters such as adrenalin. Because neurotransmitters are sensitive to the emotions one experiences, a woman's emotional life can have repercussions on her menstrual cycle.

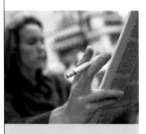

Tobacco: Public Enemy No. 1

Tobacco is not satisfie d with merely drying out skin, deepening wrinkles, destroying lungs, and ruining arteries: it attacks hormones, too. Smoking is the only factor that we can say with cer tainty advances the age of the onset of menopause. In Western societies, menopause occurs on average around the age of 50 or 51. In smokers, it arrives one to two years earlier.

The Calm after the Storm

Pre-menopause is marked by a phase of hormonal disruptions. In menopause, a new equilibrium is established.

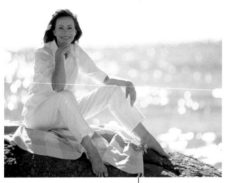

After the age of 45, 80% of women complain of irregular periods and the problems that announce the arrival of menopause.

At the time of menopause, cyclical functioning ceases with only a residual secretion of estrogens and progesterone by the adrenocorticals and the ovaries. This secretion varies greatly from one woman to the next. This is why not all women experience the same symptoms. Pre-menopause is the time before the definitive end of menstruation. At a biological level, this corresponds to a decrease in the production of progesterone. The proportion of estrogens to progesterone levels can vary from one cycle to another. Little by little, ovulation no longer occurs. This period is accompanied by disruptions in menstrual periods with a shortening or, on the contrary, a lengthening of the duration of cycles. There may be more abundant bleeding and the appearance or aggravation of pre-menstrual syndrome. There is a greater and greater space between menstrual periods, and sometimes a woman cannot be sure whether she is perhaps in the early stages of pregnancy. This is all the more problematic since the space between two cycles can be two, even three months or more. These doubts can generate a great deal of anxiety. This time period varies from 6 months to 10 years for certain women and begins on average at the age of 48. In concrete terms, 4 to 5 years before menopause, 80% of women complain of irregular periods.

The brain is at the controls

The hypothalamus is a small gland situated at the base of the brain. It manufactures the hormones that regulate the major functions controlling the human body: hunger, thirst, fatigue, body temperature, and certainly, the reproductive system. The pituitary gland directly excretes some of the hormones manufactured by the hypothalamus. The pituitary gland is located in the brain just below the hypothalamus behind the base of the nose. It also manufactures the hormones that move through the bloodstream. These hormones then stimulate the various glands situated throughout the body: the thyroid, the adrenal glands, and the ovaries. The pituitary is the "*conductor*" of the glands' "*orchestra*". It is, there f o re, subordinate to the hypothalamus and to part of the brain. It responds to the emotions by means of neuromediators. The pituitary hormones that stimulate the ovaries are FSH (follicle stimulating hormone) and LH (luteinizing hormone). The secretion of these two hormones is cyclical, and each has a peak of secretion in the middle of the cycle, which then promotes ovulation. At menopause, this cyclical secretion stops.

Mini- Glossary for better understanding

Menopause: the definitive end of menstrual periods. It can only be determined after the fact that menstruation is definitively over. Therefore, we use the term "menopause" when there have been no periods for at least one year.

Pre-menopause: the time before the definitive end of periods during which menstrual irregularities are observed.

Perimenopause: the period of time that includes pre - menopause and the year following the end of menstruation.

What are hormones for?

Estrogens and progesterone: hormones that travel throughout our entire body and help keep our daily balance..

Hormones are tiny molecules which are secreted into the blood, most often by glands. This way, they can reach all the parts of the body. When they arrive at their target organ, hormones pass through the walls of the blood vessels until they reach the cells where they must take effect.

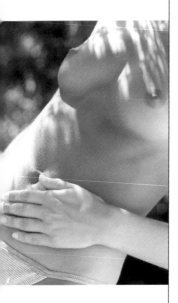

Estrogens are produced by the ovaries, placenta, and adrenal cortex. They target several organs and play an essential role in the development of female secondary sexual characteristics. Their role is:
- to help follicles and ova mature in the ovaries;
- to stimulate the proliferation of the uterine mucous membrane and increase the contractions of the uterine muscle;
- to thicken the vaginal mucous membrane and help shed epithelial cells, leading to an increased production of lactic acid, thereby lowering the vaginal pH and preventing vaginal infections;
- to increase blood coagulation;
- to retain salt and water (via estradiol), which may lead to localized edema;
- to lower cholesterol levels (via estradiol);
- to make the skin thinner and more supple.

The main role of progestatives is to allow the fertilized egg to embed itself and develop. This is the reason for their name, which means "for gestation". They are produced by the yellow body, follicle, placenta, and adrenal cortex. In order to take effect, progesterone requires the preliminary or simultaneous action of estradiol. Progesterone stimulates the growth of the uterine muscle, but reduces its activity. It transforms the uterine mucous membrane so that a fertilized egg can embed itself. With regard to the breasts, progesterone stimulates the growth of lactiferous ducts. In the kidneys, this hormone increases the excretion of salt.

Testosterone

In pre-menopausal women, testosterone is produced by the cells surrounding the ovarian follicles. At first, it is used for the production of estrogens. From the age of 20-25 up until menopause, testosterone production decreases dramatically in women. After menopause, the decrease slows down because although the follicles have disappeared, the ovaries remain active, and more DHEA (dehydroepiandrosterone) is produced by the adrenal glands and transformed into testosterone.

DHEA (dehydroepiandrosterone)

This hormone is mainly produced by the adrenal glands. Menopause does not affect its secretion. The secretion of DHEA decreases with age, independently from menopause. The decrease is the same in men.

The other important sex hormones

What happens during pre-menopause?

Progesterone levels decrease, and the body acts as if there was an excess of estrogens. The breasts increase in size and become painful, and cysts may develop. Periods become irregular; they are either further apart or closer together. More blood may be lost than usual, and hemorrhage may even occur. Premenstrual syndrome worsens.

What happens during menopause?

The ovaries have run out of ovocytes, and the cyclic secretion of sex hormones comes to an end. Periods stop, and the secretion of estrogens and progesterone is at a very low level, which varies from woman to woman. This is why every woman experiences menopause differently.

Fewer Hormones: What really changes?

The symptoms of menopause are due in part to the decrease in the hormone levels of estrogens. However, that does not explain everything: one's socio-cultural context is equally important. Scientific research continues for medicine is far from having clarified everything.

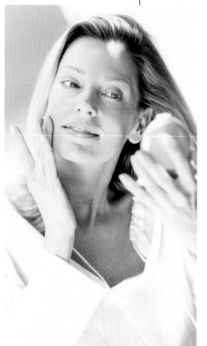

The appearance of wrinkles at menopause is not directly a result of hormone decline.

Hot Flashes:
A frequent sign

This is the annoyance of menopause most often cited by women. Hot flashes sometimes begin during pre-menopause. Around 70% of menopausal women complain of them and 30% never experience them. Hot flashes are a sensation of heat that arises rapidly, invading all or a part of the body, often accompanied by perspiration, and they can occur during the day or at night, thereby disturbing sleep. Sometimes, they are noticeable to others, which is difficult to live through. Their appearance is very uncertain and variable from one woman to another. For certain women, there will be only one or two flashes per week. For other women, they will occur several times per hour becoming a real handicap. On average, this lasts 3 years, then taper off and disappear in 5 to 8 years. Unfortunately, certain women will be bothered by hot flashes for several decades. This is often what motivates the first medical consultation for menopause. Stress, fatigue, and nervousness aggravate this phenomenon, as do the consumption of alcohol, coffee, spices, and tobacco. Physical activity and a diet rich in vitamin E decreases them.

Less supple skin

Several factors operate on the quality of the skin. The decrease in estrogens leaves the field open for the male hormones secreted by the adrenals. This explains the possible loss of hair on the forehead and the appearance of hair, especially on the upper lip.

Skin itself loses its elasticity, and its thickness decreases. Lines and wrinkles form. Brown or white spots may appear. However, these changes are not directly linked to the decrease of estrogens. Indeed, they can occur before menopause. They are certainly due to tobacco, exposure to the sun, alcohol consumption, and genetic factors. Taking estrogens, by the way, does not really improve skin quality.

Why Hot Flashes?

The hypothalamus, a small region of the brain that controls body temperature, responds to the decline of estrogens via a poorly understood mechanism. The hypothalamus reacts as though the body is overheated: it orders the central nervous system to dissipate the supposed excess heat by dilating the periphery vessels and by activating the sebaceous glands. These operations can increase skin temperature by 2.5ºC. Hot flashes persist for two to three years on average.

Disrupted Sexuality

Sexuality is an important component of health and wellbeing. At menopause, women often observe a decrease in their sexual desire. This is again, but not entirely, a consequence of hormone deficiency.

Drier Mucous Membranes

Mucous membranes are much more sensitive to hormone levels than the skin is. So, in one out of two women, menopause is accompanied by vaginal dryness that can be very embarrassing. Menopause promotes the occurrence of mycoses which are infections linked to fungi. The best known is *Candida albicans*, which causes candidiasis. Moreover, this dryness can interfere with sexual relations by causing painful intercourse. At the level of the vulva, the following changes may occur: increased scarcity of pubic hair and diminished volume of the inner and outer labia.

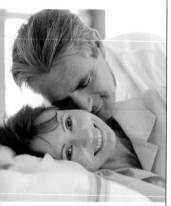

Many menopausal women complain of a decline in libido, possibly caused by insufficient levels of androgens (DHEA and testosterone.)

The uterus diminishes in volume. It atrophies, which is beneficial when there is a fibroma (benign tumour), for it will also decrease is size. If it was the cause of bleeding, it will stop.

A part of the internal mucous membrane of the bladder is very sensitive to estrogens. A too large drop in these hormones, in certain women, can induce changes that promote bladder infections. These bladder infections appear as the frequent need to urinate. There is pain during urination, such as burning or itching. Germs do not always cause these bladder infections, and urine tests are sometimes negative.

Many menopausal women say they have less sexual desire. It is not easy to say what the exact origin of this decrease of libido really is. Is it the result of hormonal decrease or of the more complex emotional difficulties of living through menopause itself? Aging is frightening. Moreover, menopause, which represents the approach of old age, is dreaded. Confidence in oneself and in one's seductive powers is put to the test. It is likely that the decrease in libido is directly linked to this problem. A long, healthy sex life is one of the best treatments for decreasing vaginal dryness.

Painful breasts

In pre-menopause, progesterone no longer battles against the action of estrogens on the breasts, and sometimes-disabling mammary pains may ensue in the second part of the cycle. Breasts enlarge and become painful. Lumps or cysts may appear and will activate the fear of cancer. An ultrasound or a mammogram will provide some reassurance.

Weight gain can generate stretch marks on the breasts. Weight loss will result in sagging, limp breasts.

A few years into menopause, the mammary gland involutes. The breasts will become softer and often smaller. They will be equally more sensitive to weight changes. Weight gain will generate stretch marks on the breasts, and weight loss will give breasts a flaccid quality. In the Western world, which exaggerates the importance of breasts as a sexual symbol, this can only accentuate a menopausal woman's feelings of uneasiness. It is best to avoid drastic weight fluctuations.

Mood Swings

The period of perimenopause is a difficult one because society so undervalues it. It is difficult to say whether the mood swings and sleep problems that ensue are directly linked to the drop in estrogens or to one's social context.

Depression, Fatigue, and Irritability

Do hormones exclusively cause these problems? This is a particular stage of life where numerous events intervene all at once. These events could explain, in and of themselves, the emotional difficulties wo m e n experience.

It is the time when children leave the nest—an overwhelming, though expected and desired, occurrence. Sometimes, marital conflicts lead to a questioning of the couple. Work pressures become more pronounced. Parents, often elderly, have health problems. The 50 - year-old woman is sandwiched in between her children's and her parents' generations. At 50, she knows she has many happy, fulfilling years of life ahead. Nevertheless, popular opinion on aging leads her to believe that this is not possible. This is also the time for profound crises of conscience on the meaning of life. The loss of loved ones often brings on this self-reflection. The investment put into work and its incessantly mounting pressures seems useless or, at the least, excessive. Putting up with 25 to 30 years of a husband's fits of anger or his lack of participation in family life becomes just too much. Some women fall prey to the demon of middle-aged lust: a more tender, more attentive companion than one's spouse can lead you to call into question years of marriage. All this and still many years ahead, that one wants to live to the fullest.

What is the actual influence of hormonal decrease on the multiple signs of this psychic and nervous fragility? It is difficult to be precise. What is certain is that hormone replacement therapy alone is often insufficient to alleviate these symptoms.

Sleep Disruptions

Sleep problems seem more frequent after 50 in both men and women, but the latter appear more vulnerable. Here once again, hormone therapy on its own is often insufficient. Sleep disruptions, ranging to complete insomnia, generate a fatigue that eventually will lead to mood swings, irritability, compensating with eating, and crying jags during the day. In order to improve this situation, a new art of living is indispensable.

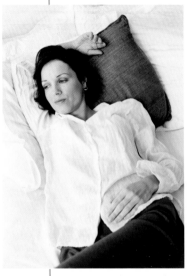

Forty percent of menopausal women complain of insomnia, fatigue, and stress.

In the general population, nearly two people in ten will, at some point, suffer from anxiety, depression, fatigue, irritability, insomnia, or stress. It is at these moments we feel especially fragile and vulnerable. In menopause, these feelings touch four in ten women.

When the Heart Suffers

Cardiovascular diseases are the leading cause of death in Canadian woman, being involved in around 34% of deaths. These diseases affect the heart or blood vessels, notably the arteries, and cause angina pectoris, heart attacks, coronary arteritis, and cerebral vascular incidents. Menopause is a period of risk.

Estrogens can't do everything

Coronary heart disease is a rather rare condition in women aged 40. However, women who suffer a heart attack at this age are more likely to die from it than men presenting the same problem. This is because estrogens cannot do everything. They cannot protect you from other risks which have been on the increase for the past 20 years in women, such as high blood pressure, high cholesterol levels, and obesity.

Blood vessel protection is no longer in effect

At the age of 40, coronary disease affects six men for every one woman. Then the ratio between men and women diminishes.

Except in very particular cases, women do not have heart attacks before menopause. Such medical troubles then become more and more frequent as age gradually increases. They then occur proportionally: the earlier the onset of menopause, the earlier the risk of heart attack. This would seem to prove that, before menopause, women's hormones perhaps protect them. The beneficial effects of estrogens could be a result, in part, of their effect on blood lipids. After menopause, one does indeed observe an increase in both total and "*bad*" cholesterol, and a decrease in "*good*" cholesterol. Moreove r, estrogens perhaps have a direct effect on artery walls by reinforcing the systems that protect against atherosclerosis.

If hormones in all likelihood play a role, other factors definitely increase the frequency of cardiovascular disease. It is more and more evident that lifestyle plays a major role.

Risk factors

Cardiovascular disease increases with the following:

- cholesterol levels ;
- blood pressure ;
- blood sugar levels ;
- homocysteine levels ;
- weight ;
- tobacco use ;
- sedentary life style ;
- stress ;
- excess refined sugar and fat

The difference in health risks between men and women before the age of 50 is perhaps also explained by women's diet, lower tobacco use, and the greater attention that women pay to their weight. In addition, with menstruation, women experience a regular elimination of blood and therefore of iron. This is perhaps beneficial as excess iron can cause heart problems. What seems more and more certain is that hormone therapy does not protect against heart disease. It is even possible that it increases the risk.

The best prevention, it seems, comes from a healthy lifestyle regimen that combines an excellent diet with relaxation. (See page 70.)

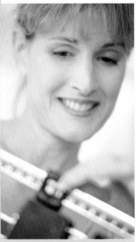

Weight: Public Enemy No.2

Fear of weight gain is justified given it is indeed observed in women around the age of 50. This weight gain occurs in women whether or not they are using a hormone treatment. There are two probable reasons for these extra pounds:

- dietary changes including an increase of sugars and fats in food intake;
- decreased physical activity.

The hormonal changes associated with menopause lead to a different distribution of fat in women. During the reproductive years, fat is stored on the thighs and hips to provide the fat stores that are quickly mobilized for pregnancies and breast-feeding. In menopause, fat moves towards the stomach! In addition, at the same time, muscle mass diminishes.

More Fragile Bones

Osteoporosis and its risks of fractures increase at menopause. It affects one out of three women after the age of 50.

Osteoporosis means porous bone. The disease is so very serious because it creates an increased susceptibility to serious fractures. Bone

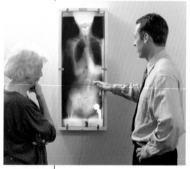

is a tissue that renews itself throughout one's lifetime. This renewal means that the destruction of old bone is succeeded by new bone's construction, achieved through the action of two types of cells: osteoclasts, which are responsible for bone destruction and osteoblasts, which ensure bone construction. All of these phenomena are dependent on hormones – including sex hormones. With advancing age, the balance between these two types of cells gradually changes.

The seriousness of osteoporosis is linked to the bone fractures that result from it.

Bone begins to weaken at the age of 35 on average. Bone loses its strength because it bonds less to calcium. In women, this bone loss is even more accentuated in the first five years of menopause. After the age of 60, bone loss continues. It is, however, much less rapid. However if, over the course of the years, bone loss is significant, then the risk of fracture increases, which is the case with osteoporosis. This disease affects one in three women after 50 and one in ten men.

Dreaded Hip Fractures

Early diagnosis is crucial but difficult since, in its beginning stages, this disease is silent and painless. When it finally announces itself, it is often already too late because a fracture is the statement. The first fractures involve the vertebrae, perhaps as a simple deformation of one or two of them. The individual's height decreases, which is not necessarily very painful. It can also appear as a fracture of a vertebra, resulting from a minor trauma or even spontaneously. These fractures can cause severe pain. The individual can no longer move. Sometimes one only becomes aware of the problem when an x-ray is taken.

Osteoporosis also affects other bones, such as the wrist and hip. Hip fracture is the most dangerous. Humans are not created equal in the face of this risk. A very important factor is the amount of bone capital built up by each individual during childhood and adolescence. In women, this capital is complete two years after the onset of the first menstrual periods. It depends especially on physical activity, but also on the intake of calcium, magnesium, potassium, and vitamin D. Physical exercise at this period must be sufficient, regular, and energetic.

Insufficient mineral supplies...

In adolescence, consuming 1,600 mg of calcium per day results in increased bone density. In fact, on average, adolescent girls ingest half of that amount. This fact would be of no consequence if they were very physically active. Alas, most are sedentary. In the same way, their intake of magnesium and potassium is often insufficient, since teenage girls avoid fruits and vegetables. As for vitamin D, most of us experience a deficiency from November to March owing to the limited hours of sunshine.

...Calcium does not explain everything

The inhabitants of Burkina Faso consume very little calcium (less than 500 mg per day) and practically no milk products, yet do not experience bone problems. Americans and Swedes devour two and a half times more dairy products, yet they are experiencing an osteoporosis epidemic. This is proof that, even if calcium is important, other environmental factors still come into play.

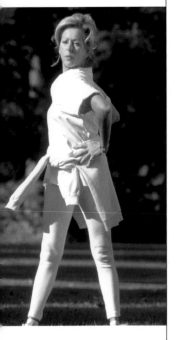

How do you know if you're at risk?

How do I know if I am at risk of developing osteoporosis or if I already have it, when I see no signs and experience no pain during the first few years of the disease?

The bone density test is a painless exam which makes it possible to measure your bone density.

This test provides an idea of your osteoporosis risk. A radiologist measures your bone density in two places: the lumbar vertebrae and the femoral head. The result consists of two figures for each measured site. The two figures are expressed compared to an average value: The T-score is obtained in comparison with the average for young women, and the Z-score is acquired in comparison with women of your age. A low value signifies osteopenia (T-score between –1 and –2.5 DS); a very low value indicates osteoporosis (T score lower than –2.5 DS). Osteopenia calls for preventative treatment, whereas osteoporosis requires curative treatment.

The bone density test may be covered by some Medicare and Medicaid programs under certain conditions (read insert). This test is very useful, as it allows you to take the necessary steps to improve the quality of your bones. In the case of diagnosed osteoporosis, a drug treatment is necessary. If you

The bone density test and Medicare /Medicaid

The test may be covered by some Medicare and Medicaid programs under certain conditions, which include the following:

once every 24 months or more often if it is medically necessary, or if you suffer from certain medical conditions;
- for men and women;

- if you are at a risk of osteoporosis.

For more detailed information, contact the Centers for Medicare and Medicaid Services.

present osteopenia, a certain number of factors depend on you. You are invited to discuss these factors with your doctor.

How can I strengthen my bones?

Throughout your life, it is vital to:

• engage in physical activities, such as walking, which "stresses" the bone matrix, or weight training, which is ideal;

• consume enough calcium (mineral water, fruit, vegetables, dairy products, or otherwise, calcium supplements);

• consume enough potassium, which allows you to fight against excess acidity in your body and to retain bone calcium (fruit, vegetables, legumes, or otherwise, potassium bicarbonate supplements);

• make sure that you get enough vitamin D (moderate sun exposure, oily fish throughout the year, and a vitamin D3 supplement from November to March).

What is harmful to bones?

Nutritional factors such as an excess intake of proteins, leading to an increased amount of waste in the urine, which depletes calcium;
Overdoing: smoking, alcohol, coffee, and sport.
Leading a sedentary lifestyle and not getting enough exercise;
Certain drugs such as corticosteroids, diuretics, antacids which contain aluminum, and excessive doses of thyroid hormones.

You have a higher risk of developing osteoporosis if:
• you are a woman;
• you are elderly;
• you are menopausal;
• you are thin or have a slight build;
• you are Caucasian (white or Asian women);
• you have already suffered an osteoporotic fracture.

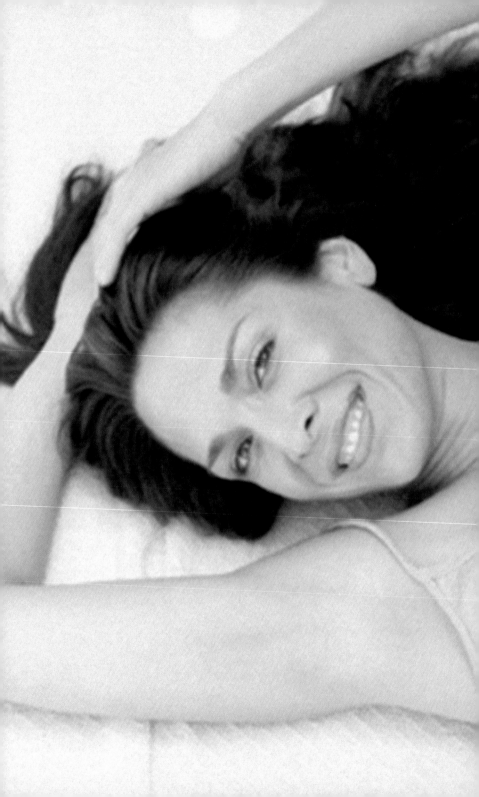

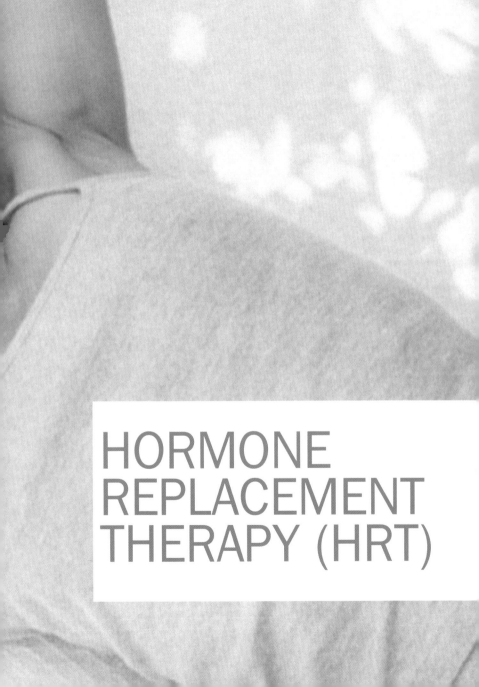

HORMONE REPLACEMENT THERAPY (HRT)

Hormone replacement therapy (HRT)

Women undergoing hormone therapy take drugs aimed at replacing the hormones which have decreased to insufficient levels.

The principle of this treatment is to consider menopause phenomena as consequences of a lack of estrogens. The treatment therefore consists of supplying the body with estrogen-like hormones, which are similar to the natural hormones no longer produced by the ovaries. At first, only estrogens were part of the treatment, but it became evident that this resulted in bleeding and even endometrial cancer (the mucous membrane that lines the uterus). Progestatives were combined with estrogens in order to protect this mucous membrane.

Estrogens used in the United States

In the United States, the estrogens used in HRT are different from the estrogens found in the contraceptive pill. The most frequently prescribed estrogen in the United States is 17 beta-estradiol, a molecule very similar to the estrogens naturally produced by women. Conjugated equine estrogens (Premarin®) – estrogens which are extracted from the urine of mares – and 17 beta-estradiol valerate (Progynova®) are more rarely prescribed. Although 17 beta-estradiol is produced chemically, it is a so-called natural molecule, as its structure is very similar to the hormones produced by the human body. This distinguishes it from ethinylestradiol, which is the molecule present in oral contraceptives.

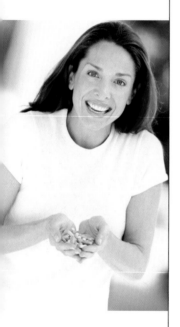

There are several ways to take estrogens. Most of the time, estrogens are taken orally, transdermally as a patch, or percutaneously as a gel. A completely new method has been developed, as the product can now be taken nasally by spraying it into each nostril once a day. Therefore, at present, women have more options than in the past. The use of patches and gels is increasing. In fact, these two modes of administration offer women more freedom while taking the product, as they can adjust the dose themselves quite finely.

Progesterone and progestatives in the United States

The combination of a progestative and estrogens is compulsory for women who have not had a hysterectomy, which renders it possible to prevent endometrial cancer. The progestative must be taken at least 12 days per month in order to counteract the harmful effects of estrogens on the uterine mucous membrane. In France, several types of molecules are used, but the main one is "natural" progesterone, which is similar to the progesterone produced by the human body. It is taken orally or percutaneously. However, in the Unites States, it is more customary to prescribe the synthesized molecule medroxyprogesterone (MPA).

Treatment with or without your period

If you wish to keep having your period, the most frequently proposed treatment is a discontinued sequential treatment. For 25 days, you will take estrogens, and during the last 12 days of treatment you will also take progestatives. During the last 5 days of the month, you will not take any medication. This is when your period will start, following discontinuation of progestatives. If you do not wish to have your period, you will take estrogens and progestatives continuously. The dose of the progestative is usually half of that used in sequential treatments

HRT worries

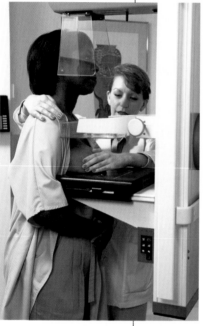

The risk of developing breast cancer is the main reason why women refuse or discontinue HRT.

What do gynecologists think of this?

Much like the uterus, the breasts are a target for hormones. Breast cancer is the most common cancer in women. Its occurrence increases with age, whether the woman has undergone HRT or not. Several studies have investigated the link between HRT and breast cancer. In July 2002, the American *Women's Health Initiative* (WHI) study made it possible to determine the risk of cancer with a type of HRT rarely used in France. Other studies, particularly those that were conducted on a large number of English women (*the Million Women Study*) and French women (the E3N study) provided further information.

In 2007, gynecologists agreed that HRT, which prolongs the exposure to estrogens, increases the breast cancer risk in HRT-treated women as compared to non-treated women. HRT which combines estrogens and a progestative increases the risk of breast cancer. As for estrogen-only HRT, it appears that the risk does not increase. It has been estimated that among 100,000 women at the peak of HRT use (years 2000 – 2002), between 35 and 55 cases of breast cancer can be ascribed to HRT. Note that

The risk of breast cancer increases:

• with age;
• if there is a family history of breast cancer in your mother, sister, or daughter;
• if you have already had breast disease;
• with certain hormonal factors, such as having had your first period at an early age, having your first pregnancy or menopause at a late age, and undergoing estrogen-only HRT.

although it is true that the occurrence of breast cancer is on the rise, the death rate for this cancer has not increased. This shows that the disease is diagnosed at an earlier stage and is treated more effectively.

Women's opinions

Today, many women in their 50s know someone who has been treated for breast cancer. In 2009 in the USA, approximately 192,000 new cases were diagnosed. This type of cancer frightens women, and the fact that HRT increases their risk discourages them from this treatment, even though the risk is tiny. The lack of clarity in publications causes them to be even more suspicious. Women think that the risk is played down or that the role of HRT is lost among the other points made.

Despite the reassurance of gynecologists and pharmaceutical companies, women do not want to take risks. After all, it is true that there is a risk.

Progesterone is called into question

In November 2004, Dr Françoise Clavel-Chapelon (from the Gustave Roussy Institute in Villejuif) published the results from the sole French study on the risk of breast cancer linked to HRT: the **E3N study.** According to this study, women who were given a combination of estrogens and a synthesized progestative had a 40% higher risk of developing breast cancer than those who did not undergo HRT. Women who were given a combination of estrogens and natural progesterone did not display an increased risk.

Cancer: the first cause of death in men and the second in women

Although the exact causes of cancer in general are not yet known, certain risk factors have been clearly identified:
• smoking, undoubtedly the worst one of them all;
• alcohol;
• the sun;
• hormones (in the case of hormone-dependent cancers such as breast cancer and endometrial cancer in women, and prostate cancer in men);
• unbalanced diet with too much animal fat and refined sugar

Does HRT prevent cardiovascular diseases?

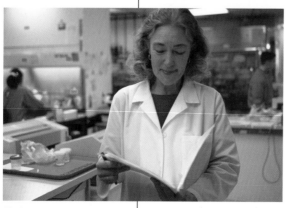

The American WHI study was discontinued in July 2002 due to the excessive occurrence of cardiovascular disease in women undergoing hormone treatment.

At least this is what we used to believe before a large American study caused confusion.

While it is recognized that HRT (slightly) increases the risk of breast cancer, only a few months ago, doctors still believed that this risk was compensated by the expected benefits in terms of cardiovascular prevention. As these diseases are two to three times more common in women older than 50, this statement bore a lot of weight.

The latest research results bear disappointment

The *Women's Health Initiative (WHI)* study is an American study which was initiated in 1997 in order to evaluate the effects of standard American HRT on cardiovascular health and the risk of cancer. The study compared HRT to a placebo. While researchers expected to find fewer heart attacks and strokes in the group receiving estrogens and progesterone, the opposite came true. The study was designed to continue until 2005, but had to be discontinued in 2002. However, you should note that the doses, molecules, and modes of administration used differed from those used for HRT in many countries. This did not lessen the concerns brought about by the WHI study, which caused the arguments for a possible beneficial effect of HRT on the cardiovascular system to be discounted.

HRT and mistrust

According to the North American Menopause Society, in 2000, 37.5 million American women began menopause or were already menopausal. According to IMS Health, a health information company, in 2008, approximately 42 million prescriptions for HRT were dispensed, which is a decrease of 6.2% from around 45 million during the previous year. It seems that HRT is putting women off and worrying them, and the early discontinuation of the WHI study has increased these concerns.

Hormones and vessels

Data from the American WHI study suggests that HRT increases the risk of cardiovascular diseases. Among 1,000 women treated over 10 years, there are apparently seven additional heart attack cases, eight additional cases of stroke, and eight additional cases of pulmonary embolism.

The risk of venous thrombosis may increase

The number of venous thrombosis cases increases after menopause. The ESTHER study, which was conducted between 1999 and 2004, particularly analyzed the effect of HRT on this disease in menopausal women aged 45 to 75. The results showed that all depends on the type of HRT used. The risk automatically increases if the estrogen is taken orally, whether in combination with a progestative or not. However, if the estrogen is taken transdermally (as a patch), the risk directly depends on the associated progestative molecule. The risk increases if a norpregnane-type progestative is being used, whereas the risk is the same as that for untreated women if natural micronized progesterone or a pregnane-type progestative is taken. Note that other personal risk factors, such as obesity, may increase the harmful effects of estrogens taken orally.

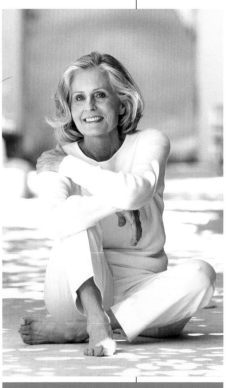

When hormones are back

HRT undeniably improves the quality of life of women who are highly inconvenienced by menopause. It also prevents osteoporosis.

A new quality of life

HRT has remarkable effects on all the inconveniences related to menopause. It improves women's lives in a significant way:

- Hot flashes disappear (in more than 85% of cases), most frequently from the first month onward;
- Night sweats decrease;
- The skin becomes suppler;
- Vaginal dryness improves;
- Urinary tract infections decrease;
- Mood, sleep, and general balance problems improve, probably because HRT alleviates menopause symptoms.

What HRT does not do

It does not prevent skin ageing.
It does not directly improve the libido!
It does not improve stress incontinence or urge incontinence.
It does not prevent muscle wasting.
It does not eliminate excess fat.
It does not prevent cognitive problems.

With regard to bones, HRT prevents spinal fractures if it is administrated as soon as menopause sets in. It slows the progression of vertebral osteoporosis if it is already present. HRT is undoubtedly useful for preventing hip fractures. It is necessary to continue the treatment for a long time, most often beyond the age of 80. The problem is that undergoing this treatment over a long period of time also increases the harmful effects. This is the dilemma facing menopausal women.

In the WHI study, HRT also decreased the risk of **colorectal cancer.** For 1,000 women treated for 10 years, HRT prevented six cases of colorectal cancer. Yet, at present, the studies conducted in France do not make it possible to prove that "French" HRT protects against cancer.

Does HRT make you gain weight?

Some women complain that they gain weight during menopause. There are several explanations for this: a sedentary lifestyle, snacking as compensation, and most definitely, the decrease in hormones.

Weight increases with age, while muscle mass decreases and gives way to fat. The decrease in estrogens is responsible for this, but it is not the only factor. The growth hormone (GH), testosterone, and DHEA, which normally act against fat storage, are also to blame. Moreover, fats are distributed in different ways and are usually stored around the abdominal area. The question is what effect does HRT have on the figure? Studies suggest that appropriately-dosed HRT does not increase body weight. A study on 671 women between the ages of 65 and 94 showed that women undergoing hormone therapy were slimmer than those who did not. It is true that some women are particularly sensitive to hormones and will therefore feel "bloated". In this case, it would be appropriate to reduce the estrogen dose.

HRT and Alzheimer's disease

Contrary to our hopes, there is no proof today that HRT prevents Alzheimer's disease. The opposite could even be true, as HRT might increase the risk of dementia in women older than 65.

Shumaker SA: *Estrogen plus progestin and the incidence of dementia and mild cognitive impairment in postmenopausal women: The Women's Health Initiative Memory Study (WHIMS). JAMA 2003, 289, 2651-2662.*

Contraindications of HRT

Contra-indications are linked to possible side effects of estrogens.

Absolute contra-indications

A woman should not undergo HRT:
- if she suffers from a type of hormone-dependant cancer such as breast cancer, endometrial cancer, or ovarian cancer;
- if she has a history of venous or arterial thrombosis or embolism (e.g., pulmonary embolism, phlebitis, angina pectoris, heart attack, or stroke);
- if she has heart disease presenting a risk of embolism;
- if she has had a disease affecting the eyes' blood vessels;
- if she has high levels of triglycerides in the blood.

Ladies, get informed!

It is essential for women to be sufficiently informed in order to make the correct choice in full knowledge of the facts. Their health depends on it! In a context where the law requires doctors to inform the patients and respect their choices, it is vital that women insist that their doctors give them scientific arguments for and against different types of treatment. While knowing the facts, it is up to the women themselves to choose what would suit them best.

Relative contra-indications

Currently, there is some dispute about the relative contra-indications, which are the following:
- fibrocystic breast disease;
- interstitial fibroma (i.e., in the uterine wall) or subserous fibroma;
- bleeding fibroma, as the added amount of hormones may increase bleeding;
- endometriosis;
- non-insulin dependant diabetes;
- a history of serious migraines.

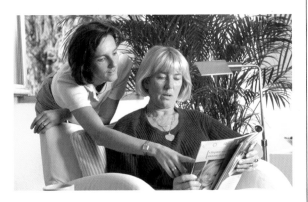

For some doctors, these contra-indications prohibit HRT. Others consider that the beneficial effects of HRT in terms of osteoporosis prevention outweigh the risks.

Precautions

Before starting HRT, arterial hypertension must be treated, and excessive cholesterol levels in the blood must be decreased. Women should not smoke in general, but abstaining from tobacco is even more important during HRT, as the risks of phlebitis and pulmonary embolism become even higher.

It seems that it is very difficult today to have clear information about the side effects of HRT. When one study indicates risks, another study reveals that these risks are not the same for all types of HRT. New scientific studies are being conducted, and while we await the results, let us rather err on the side of caution.

Alternative to HRT:
SERM and SAS

SERMs are prescribed for preventing and treating osteoporosis. The SAS relieve hot flashes and other symptoms of menopause.

Estrogens, mainly produced in the ovaries, reach the blood and are then distributed throughout the entire body. Some cells have a high affinity for these molecules, as they contain estrogen-specific receptors. There are two receptor types: the alpha type, which is found in the breast, uterus, and liver cells, and the beta type, which is mainly found in the bones, cardiovascular system, and ovaries.

There are drugs that act specifically on these receptors: the SERM (*Selective Estrogen Receptor Modulators*), *raloxifen being at the head of this group of drugs* (Evista®, Optruma®). These molecules are simultaneously estrogen antagonists and agonists. In other words, they act like estrogens (agonistic action), and they also inhibit the action of estrogens by binding themselves to the estrogen receptors (antagonistic action). The type of action depends on the type of targeted tissue.

A positive effect on bones

Raloxifen has a positive effect on bones, which is the reason why it is recommended for preventing and treating vertebral osteoporosis in women vulnerable to osteoporosis. Studies showed that the occurrence of breast

Medication for bones

Apart from raloxifen, there are other drugs that strengthen bones and prevent fractures:
- biphosphonates such as alendronate (Fosamax) and risedronate (Actonel), which reduce bone resorption and have to be taken once a week only;
- teriparatide (Forsteo), an analogue of parathormone, which helps produce bone tissue and significantly reduces the risk of vertebral fracture;
- strontium ranelate (Protelos), which inhibits osteoclasts that destroy bone tissue, stimulates osteoblasts that build bone tissue, and reduces the risk of vertebral and hip fractures. This drug is not yet available in the United States.

cancer is reduced, essentially for tumors which carry estrogen receptors. The drug has no harmful effects on the endometrium. However, this drug has only recently been put on the market, and we should therefore be cautious.

For the same reasons, its contra-indications are identical to those of HRT. The product does not have any effect on hot flashes.

SAS

SAS, which stands for "selective action steroid", are currently represented by only one molecule, tibolone (Livial®). This is a synthesized steroid with weak estrogenic, progestative, and androgenic properties.

Tibolone acts on hot flashes, vaginal dryness, and sleep and mood disturbances. Additionally, this product improves libido. Unfortunately, tibolone increases the risk of endometrial cancer, as the "Million Women" study demonstrated. It also 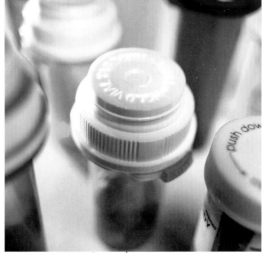 increases the risk of breast cancer and stroke. Therefore, it has the same contra-indications as HRT. As far as the bones are concerned, tibolone decreases bone loss, but there is not enough data available to date to suggest that it should be used as a preventive or curative treatment for osteoporosis.

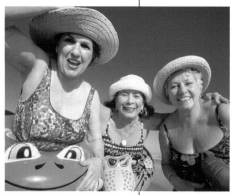

DHEA: Hormone of youth?

This a very controversial product: Should one take it or not?

DHEA may be prescribed by doctors and dispensed by pharmacists in Europe, but is freely available in the United States. With a prescription, it is also possible to buy it in other countries.

DHEA (dehydroepiandrosterone) is a weak steroidal hormone produced by the adrenal glands. It circulates in the blood and body in the form of DHEA sulfate, and transforms itself into estrogens and testosterone. Its exacts role is still unknown. It is found in the brain, adrenal glands, ovaries, testes, fat tissue, skin, and blood. Just before puberty sets in, DHEA is produced in large quantities. From the age of 30, its production decreases steadily, and at the age of 70, the quantity produced is only 20% of that which was synthesized at the age of 20. In the United States, the DHEA boom began in the 1980s. Today, only the United States, where it is freely available, considers it to be a dietary supplement. In France, it is considered to be a drug and cannot be bought without a prescription.

What does the research show?

A lot of research has been done on DHEA. France's Prof. Étienne-Émile Baulieu is the most active DHEA researcher. His research showed that women over 70 benefit the most from this product. DHEA improves bone metabolism and decreases osteoporosis. But that is not the only positive effect. DHEA gives women a youth boost, as it improves skin hydration, physical condition, mood, and libido. Numerous studies have been conducted, but unfortunately, almost all of them only focus on a small number of people. To make conclusions based on these studies would be very premature, as they only represent interesting lines of thought.

Here are some details:

• Applying a cream containing 10% of DHEA improved the bone strength of 14 women aged 60. This does not mean that we can conclude that DHEA is an anti-osteoporotic treatment!

• Low DHEA blood levels correlate with a risk of depression. But we cannot conclude that DHEA is an antidepressant!

• Taking DHEA improves morale and libido in women after menopause. However, this does not mean that DHEA is an aphrodisiac.

DHEA is not harmless

It is important not to forget that DHEA is a semi-synthetic hormone. It can transform itself into estrogen or testosterone in the body. There are therefore some possible side effects. Much like estrogens, it can, in theory, contribute to the development of hormone-dependent cancer s uch as breast cancer and endometrial cancer. Similarly to testosterone, DHEA can cause acne and hirsutism. It may also cause the voice to become lower, decrease the levels of good cholesterol, induce insulin resistance, and rise bl ood pressure. The other, less severe, side effects include abdominal pain, fatigue, headaches, and nasal congestion. DHEA is therefore completely contra-indicated for persons who have or have had a hormone-dependent cancer. In addition, those who suffer from liver or kidney dysfunction should not take this drug. Let us rather wait for the studies before consuming DHEA.

What about natural DHEA?

One can find "natural" DHEA in stores. In general, these are yam, soy, and clover extracts. While these products are useful as phytoestrogens or phytoprogesterone, they do not in any way increase DHEA levels in the blood. **There is no natural DHEA!**

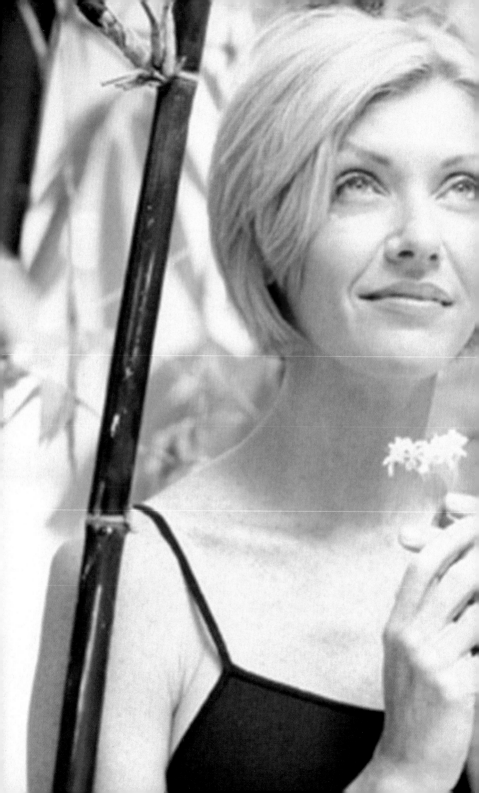

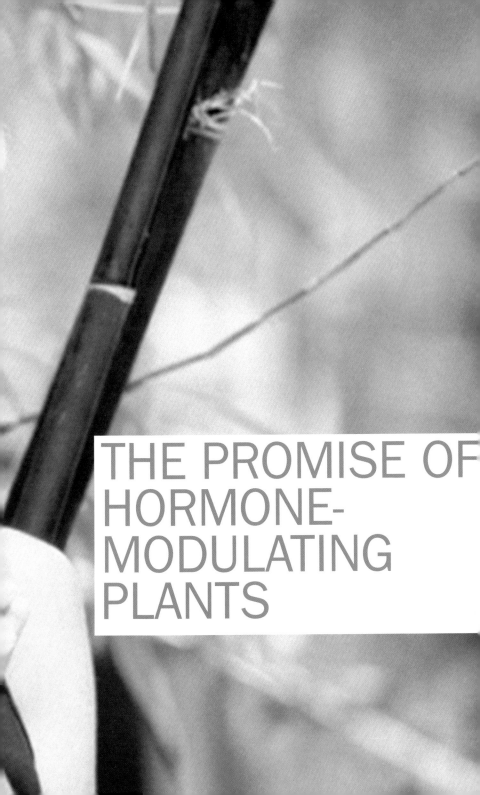

THE PROMISE OF HORMONE-MODULATING PLANTS

Phytoestrogens

Plants naturally produce substances that mimic estrogens when ingested. They are called phytoestrogens or plant estrogens. Nowadays these molecules hold a special place in the therapeutic arsenal of menopause.

History of a discovery

At the beginning of the 1940s, a mysterious infertility epidemic among sheep narrowly missed decimating flocks of sheep in Southeast Australia. Desperate and on the verge of ruin, farmers successively put the blame on genetic mutations, radiation, and pesticides. They had to wait until 1946 for the Australian Agriculture Ministry to identify the culprit, a variety of clover (Trifolium subterraneum) that the sheep farmers had planted several years earlier. No one suspected that this plant naturally manufactured significant quantities (5% of its dry weight) of substances that mimic female hormones when ingested. These substances are known as phytoestrogens. In the 1950s, two of the substances that belong to the isoflavone family, genistein and daidzein, were isolated. A great many plants, including clover and soy, synthesize these substances. The significance of these molecules for the health and wellbeing of menopausal women was first suspected following epidemiological observations in Asian countries. Indeed, Asian women suffer very little from hot flashes. Fewer than 25% of Japanese and Chinese women complain of them as opposed to 85% of North American and 75% of European women. Moreover, Asian women have far less cardiovascular disease, breast cancer, and osteoporosis. Researchers attempted to discover what in the lifestyle of Asian women could explain this advantage. They also noticed that when these women emigrated to the United States, for example, and adopted a Western lifestyle, they gradually were affected by the same problems as Western women. The researchers concluded that this difference was most likely a result of the Asian women's diet and, in particular, of their substantial consumption of soy, the food richest in phytoestrogens.

Soy: the noble food

The oldest book of the Chinese pharmacopeia, the *Shen Nong Ben Cao,* already mentioned soy around 2700 B.C. Tofu produced from soy has been a fundamental part of the Chinese diet for the past 4 millennia. Between the 2nd and the 7th century, Buddhist monks introduced it to Japan and Korea. At the Chinese emperor's court, tofu was recognized as a noble food. In Asian countries, soy has been a basic part of the diet for many centuries, as soy proteins constitute 20 to 60% of all proteins consumed.

Where are phytoestrogens found?

Phytoestrogens are found in more than 600 plants. They are divided into three large families:

• isoflavones, which are mostly found in legumes such as soybeans, but also chickpeas, green beans, tea, etc.;

• lignans from whole grains, oily grains (flaxseed; olives; sunflower seeds), flageolets, lentils, cherries, apples, pears, grapefruit, garlic, etc.

• coumestans, whose structure resembles that of isoflavones and which are found in alfalfa and especially in soybean sprouts.

How Phytoestrogens work

The majority of scientific studies relating to phytoestrogens have been conducted on soy and soy isoflavones.

Highly Active Substances

When soy isoflavones reach the stomach, they are hydrolyzed. They then pass to the intestine where they are transformed by intestinal bacteria into the active substances genistein and daidzein. Many parameters affect this transformation, which explains the varying blood levels of these substances observed among individuals. These parameters include intestinal flora quality, transit speed, and pH level. Of the two substances, genistein has been studied the most to date.

The two faces of isoflavones

Isoflavones have a chemical structure similar to that of estrogens. Because of this resemblance, these molecules can link to the same receptors, but they have varied effects according to the organs targeted. Indeed, isoflavones seem to behave like Selective Estrogen Receptor Modulators (SERMs).

Soy: a fundamental part of the Asian diet

In Asia, soy is transformed into soy milk and tofu but also into fermented soy, in the form of miso, tempeh, soy sauce, etc. Fermented soy contains many isoflavones. Tofu and soy milk only contain genisteine and daidzeine.

What amounts of isoflavones are found in the Western diet?

It is estimated that no more than 5mg of isoflavones are included in the Western diet per day, while in Asian populations, 25 to 45mg of isoflavones are consumed daily. The Japanese consume the most, as they eat approximately 200mg of soy-based products daily. Some experts consider that the consumption of isoflavones may even reach 250mg per day in some Asian populations.

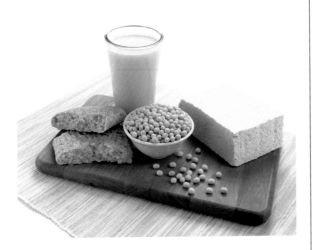

Clarification: Researchers recently discovered that two types of estrogen receptors exist, alpha-receptors and beta-receptors, and that their distribution varies according to tissue type. Isoflavones have six times greater affinity for beta-receptors than for alphareceptors. Therefore, isoflavones have an estrogenic effect on certain tissues (brain, bones, lung, vessels, bladder…) and anti-estrogenic effects on others (ovary, breast, uterus…).

Effects vary

If the distribution of the receptors varies according to the tissues, the density of these receptors also varies from one woman to another. This could explain the inconsistent effectiveness of soy isoflavones.

Average isoflavone content
μg/100g of dry weight

Soybeans	40,000 to 200,000
Peanuts	120
Chickpeas	80 to 400
Lentils	10 to 30
Barley	22
Broccoli	15
Cauliflower	15

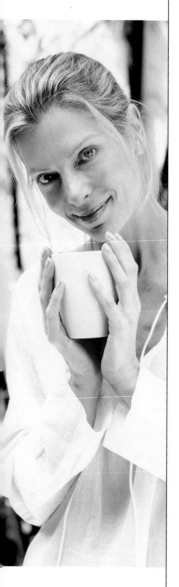

The Benefits of Soy Extracts

Since the discovery of the estrogenic activity of isoflavones, research has been simmering with excitement. Taken complementary to diet, soy extracts diminish hot flashes. In addition, the benefits do not stop there.

Women can now obtain from their pharmacists soy-based, isoflavone-rich supplements that will help them overcome the chaotic period of menopause.

Proven effectiveness for hot flashes

Seven double-blind clinical studies tested the effectiveness of soy extracts in menopausal women. Six clearly proved the effectiveness of isoflavones taken complementary to diet. Six clearly proved the effectiveness of isoflavones taken complementary to diet. For the Professor Mark Messina (Loma Linda University), who is one of the best specialist of soy benefits on health, the isoflavones effects on hot flashes are positive. Among women suffering debilitating hot flashes, researchers observed that a daily dose of stan-

The Strongest Bones in the World

The Okinawa archipelago is a group of 44 islands that extend from Japan to Taiwan. In comparison with other Japanese women, who already experience a great health advantage, the women of Okinawa have 20% fewer hip fractures. Studies have shown that Japanese women begin to lose calcium from the age of 40 and Japanese men, from the age of 50, whereas this decline occurs much later in Okinawa. While the Japanese overall and the residents of Okinawa consume essentially the same quantity of isoflavones, the island dwellers are more physically active and so get a great deal more vitamin D.

dardized soy extract containing 70 mg of isoflavones resulted in a decrease of 65% of symptoms as opposed to only 28% in the group that received a placebo. In June 2001, the American College of Obstetricians and Gynecologists (ACOG) officially recognized the importance of phytoestrogens in the short-term treatment of vasomotor problems.

Stronger Bones: The Asians' Secret

Epidemiological studies have made it possible to certify that the incidence of hip fractures is much lower in Asia than in the West. Japanese women have a fracture risk 40% lower than that of American women. Are phytoestrogens at the origin of the sturdiness of Asian women's bones? This is what researchers are trying to understand. After several promising trials on animal models (ovariotomized rats), the first human trials are now underway. Two recently published studies point to promising prospects. (See sidebar.)

How can we explain this phenomenon?

Isoflavones might be able to intervene in the process of bone restructuring because of their estrogenic action. They possibly stimulate the activity of osteoblasts and simultaneously inhibit bone resorption. This seems to be confirmed by the fact that the slowing of bone loss essentially appears at the level of the spinal column. Indeed, vertebrae consist of a large proportion of spongy bone, the bone tissue that renews itself the most quickly, and which is the most sensitive to estrogens.

Soy and Bone Health: An Encouraging Study

Researchers at the University of Illinois in the U.S. studied the influence of soy-isoflavone supplements on bone loss in menopausal women. Sixtysi women were divided at random into three groups. Each group consumed 40 grams of soy proteins daily containing, respectively, 45 mg of isoflavones, 90 mg, or a casein placebo. Only the group that received 90 mg of isoflavones per day experienced a significant increase in the mass and bone density of their lumbar ver tebrae at the end of 24 weeks. The researchers obser ved no effect on the femur.

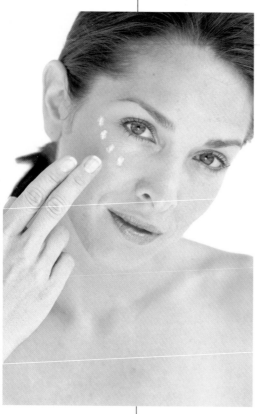

Soy Prevents Serious Chronic Illness

What emerges from the body of research is that women who eat soy or who take it in the form of a food supplement have a lower risk of cardio-vascular disease and cancer.

In terms of cardiovascular health, Asians are again better off than we are in the West. Certainly, their diet is rich in vegetable fibre and contains few saturated fats, which is already advantageous, but the special role of soy in its protective capabilities is also very seriously considered.

Studies carried out on animals and humans demonstrate that isoflavones have an effect on blood lipids and decrease the risk of cardio-vascular diseases.

They significantly reduce "bad cholesterol" (LDL) and triglycerides, and increase "good cholesterol" (HDL). Because of their antioxidant properties, isoflavones also protect cholesterol from free radical attacks. They oppose the formation of arterial plaque —the cause of infarctions— by direct action on the vascular wall.

Finally, a recent study shows that soy decreases homocysteine, a by-product of dietary protein that is toxic to arteries. These benefits appear after a quantity of 50 mg of isoflavo n e s, that is to say 25 g of soy proteins or more per day. The U.S. Food and Drug Administration

Safe, reliable compounds

As opposed to HRT, isoflavones appear to present no danger to the breasts, endometrium, and ovaries. Moreover, for Professor Petra Peeters (University of Utrecht, the Netherlands), one of the world's leading specialists, phytoestrogens a re devoid of toxicity to humans.

Isoflavones on the skin

Studies have shown that applying a cream containing soy isoflavones improves the skin's protection against oxidants.

(FDA) recently allowed manufacturers of soy-based foods to indicate on their packaging that a diet that includes soy can decrease the risk of cardio-vascular disease.

Prevention of breast, ovarian, and endometrial cancers

Isoflavones have given rise to a great deal of hope in the prevention of hormone-dependent cancers. Asian women, whose diet is rich in phytoestrogens, have six times fewer breast cancers than Western women do.

Their risk of these cancers increases when they emigrate to the United States.

Women of Japanese origin born in the U.S. have a level of risk almost identical to American women. Several studies have found weaker concentrations of lignans and isoflavones in the urine of patients with breast cancer compared to women in good health.

In vitro studies have effectively demonstrated a protective effect, but it is too soon to provide conclusive answers.

Researchers explain this protection by the tissue-selective effects of isoflavones.

The many forms of soy

Soy milk is made from soybeans that are boiled. Next, the mixture is ground and finally filtered.
Soy milk is the filtrate obtained from this process.

Tonyu is soy milk, made exclusively from whole soybeans and not from isolates or soy flour and containing a minimum protein content of 36g/l.

Tofu is made by adding a fermenting agent to soy milk, which causes it to curdle. It is then
pressed into blocks. Tofu is very bland and must be p re p a re d in dishes and seasoned.

Miso is a fermented paste made from yellow soy and is very salty. It is used as the base for
Japanese miso soup.

Tempeh is fermented yellow soybeans, sometimes with coconut.

Soya sauce is also made from fermented soy. The best soya sauce is a salty liquid that requires
six to seven years of maturation.

Tamari is also salty, fermented soy sauce.

Soybeans can also be prepared and used as you would lentils or peas.

Do Isoflavones Protect against Other Cancers?

Research studies are growing in number and have found several very interesting effects of isoflavones.

Studies generate hope

Researchers have carried out in vitro laboratory studies on human and animal cells. They show that:
- phytohormones are antioxidants ;
- they inhibit the vascularization of tumours, the flow of blood to a tumour (angiogenesis) ;
- they induce the death of cancerous cells by apoptosis ;

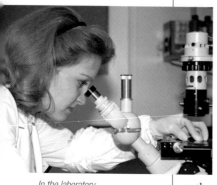

In the laboratory, phytoestrogens prevent small tumours from developing.

- they inhibit a special enzyme called aromatase, which normally transforms androgens into estrogens at the level of the mammary gland;
- they inhibit other enzymes that are implicated in the spontaneous generation of cancerous cells ;
- they inhibit the proliferation of tumoural cells in liver and breast cancers, melanomas, and in leukaemic cells ;

Overall, phytohormones prevent the development of cancer cells in tissue cultures. These different effects vary according to the dosages used.

In animals, phytohormones have a preventative effect against certain cancers: colon, chemo-induced, liver, mammary gland, and prostate cancers. The consumption of soy prevents the growth of prostate, breast, and colon tumours. In humans, epidemiological studies show that soy consumption is associated with a lower risk of lung cancer, leukaemia, and prostate cancer.

A serious alternative to HRT

Overall, soy isoflavones provide numerous benefits for the health and well-being of women at menopause. From now on, they constitute a genuine alternative for women who either cannot or do not wish to undergo HRT.

To optimize the effectiveness of these products, it is important to have healthy intestinal flora, which necessitates good dietary habits. Women will feel the first effects after ingesting from 50 mg onwards of soy isoflavones per day. To achieve effects that are even more complete, particularly in the areas of bone and cardiovascular health, they can increase the daily dosage without risk to a consumption of between 80 and 100 mg per day.

A More-than-complete Food

Soy contains more that just isoflavones. It is rich in proteins that contain the amino acids essential to humans, in the same way as the proteins in meat, fish, eggs, and milk products do. Among plants, only quinoa is comparable. It can therefore replace meat. Moreover, soy contains few lipids, and those it does are beneficial since they are rich in omega-3 unsaturated fatty acids. These fatty acids help protect against cardiovascular diseases. Soy also contains phospholipids, which manufacture chemical messages used by the brain for the memory.

The most famous phytoprogesterones

Several plants seem to have an effect which resembles that of progesterone, in other words, they are progesterone-like. The chaste tree berry is one of them, but the most famous example is the yam, or wild yam.

The overrated reputation of yams

The wild *yam*, whose botanical name is *Dioscorea villosa*, originally comes from Mexico. The Discoreaceae family includes more than 300 plants. Only some of them are used, either for dietary needs or for their medicinal properties. The wild yam was already used by the Aztecs for treating rheumatism and was applied topically as a way of relieving pain. In Central America, it was used for menstrual and ovarian problems and for facilitating labor.

In the 20th century, a very interesting molecule was extracted from it: diosgenine. By a chemical process, diosgenine can be transformed into progesterone. It was thanks to this molecule that it became possible to industrially produce progesterone, and around the 1960s, to produce the first female oral contraceptive. A little later, another chemical process was discovered that made it possible to transform progesterone into cortisone.

Unfortunately, the diosgenine found in yams does not increase progesterone or DHEA levels in the blood when it is ingested. Today, controlled studies do not show any evidence that yams are useful during menopause, except for the fact that they have an antioxidant effect. One must be very careful when taking yam tablets, as certain manufacturers add progesterone to them.

You can also find yam-based creams on the market, which are proposed as a way of re-establishing your hormonal balance. To this day, no study conducted on women has proved this type of effect. In fact, studies show that the yam has a weak estrogen-like action. It is traditionally used for spasms, aerophagy, colic, morning sickness, and pain resulting from inflammation.

Yams and pre-menopause

While the term "natural progesterone" is incorrect when referring to yams, other plants actually do have a progesterone-like action. This is true for the chaste tree berry, or *Vitex agnus castus.*

The chaste tree berry has been used since Hippocrates's time (450 B.C.) for regulating menstrual problems, facilitating the delivery of the placenta, and stimulating lactation. Its action is particularly interesting in pre-menopause, as, like progesterone, it reduces breast pain. It also reduces edema and helps regulate the menstrual cycle. It has a beneficial effect on headaches, constipation, and mood swings during this period.

In the blood, it acts efficiently on the levels of certain hormones and has progesterone-like effects. It alleviates premenstrual syndrome and is particularly recommended during pre-menopause.

Directions for use: It must be taken for 3 months, either in the form of capsules or as a mother tincture. In the latter case, one should take 40 drops per day.

Chaste tree berry: Emblem of the Vestal Virgins of Ancient Rome

Pliny the Elder recommended the chaste tree berry for men affected by violent sexual d e s i res. Monks used it in cooking, as its peppery taste spiced up plain food, while at the same time diminished libido! This is why it is also called Monk's pepper and has become a symbol of chastity.

The phyto-progesterones on which you can rely

The chaste tree berry is not the only plant which behaves like a progestative. Here is a detailed look at beneficial plants.

Common yarrow (Achillea millefolium)

Achilles gave his name to this plant because he used it to his treat wounded soldiers. This plant is found throughout the Northern hemisphere.

From a gynecological perspective, common yarrow regulates the menstrual cycle, decreases bleeding, and relieves period pain.

Directions for use: From June to October, use the flowery tips. In order to stop bleeding, make a brew of three flowery tips in a cup of tea, boil for 3 minutes, and then strain. For treating irregular periods and period

Magnesium: an essential mineral

Magnesium is essential during the treatment of irregular periods and period problems, as a magnesium deficiency could aggravate the symptoms. Magnesium has sedative properties. It plays a role in muscle contraction, heartbeat regulation, nerve impulse transmission, and energy storage and use. Some researchers observed lower magnesium levels in the blood in women suffering from premenstrual syndrome. Another study showed that taking a magnesium supplement every day (360mg) could improve your mood during this critical time in your cycle.

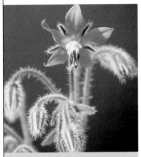

pain, you can use a mother tincture. Take 20 to 50 drops per day. The Chinese use the stems of dried common yarrow when they consult the I Ching, a divination book.

Lady's mantle (Alchemilla vulgaris)

Originally from Europe, this plant is picked in summer. Its name *Alchemilla* stems from the fact that it fascinated alchemists. Lady's mantle is also used for its anti-hemorrhaging properties in war injuries.

From a gynecological point of view, the plant regulates the menstrual cycle and relieves period pain. It is useful for fibroma and endometriosis.

Directions for use: Use the mother tincture for regulating your periods and relieving period pain. Take 20 to 50 drops per day.

Rough bindweed (Smilax aspera)

This plant grows in the temperate regions of Asia and Australia. The root of this plant is used for skin problems such as eczema and psoriasis, but it is also useful from a gynecological perspective, as, like the previous plants, it stimulates the production of progesterone. It is therefore indicated for premenstrual syndrome and problems related to pre-menopause.

Directions for use: Take 20 to 50 drops of a mother tincture per day.

Other Useful Plants for Pre- menopause

Verbena officinalis, gromwell, comfrey, melissa officinalis (lemon balm), marjoram, rosemary, wild thyme, thyme, bugloss, and borage.

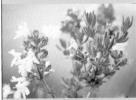

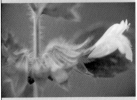

From top to bottom: borage, thyme, lemon balm

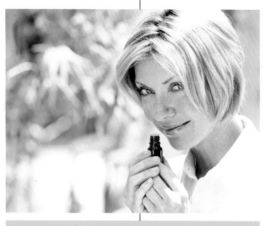

Aromatherapy
the essence of the plant

Essential oils extracted from plants also have a very useful effect, which complements phytotherapy.

Essential oils are very active and must be kept out of children's reach. Some of them can irritate the skin and should therefore be used with caution. The quantity that should be absorbed is minimal: Do not exceed seven drops per day if you are self-medicating.

The letters E.O. feature after the name of the plant if it is an essential oil.

The quintessence of plants

Essential oils are obtained through the distillation of plants, which leaves us with the quintessence of plants. They are at the same time oils (soluble in fats or lipophiles) and essences (soluble in water, alcohol, or hydrophiles). Their double solubility enables them to circulate in all parts of the body and be very effective. However, you should be careful when using these oils. Only take them as your phytotherapy specialist or specialized pharmacist recommends.

Basil E.O. (Ocimum basilicum)

This oil is particularly effective for premenstrual syndrome during pre-menopause.
It is used over a short period of time: Take two drops three times a day for 2 to 3 days during period pain. You can also mix it with massage oil and rub it onto your abdomen two to three times a day.

Mediterranean Cypress H.E. (Cupressus sempervirens)

This oil is very helpful if you suffer from period pain. It also improves your mood before and during your period.

It stimulates venous circulation and fights nervous fatigue. Do not use this oil if you have hormone-dependant cancer or mastosis. Use it over a short period of time: two drops three times a day for 2 to 3 days during period pain.

Tarragon E.O. (Artemisia dracunculus)

Tarragon essential oil has the same indications as the two previous oils and is used in the same way. These three oils can also be used at the same times as soon as premenstrual syndrome sets in. Take a drop of each oil four times a day for the first 2 days of your period.

Chamomile E.O. (Ormenis multiple)

This oil has a relaxing effect, helps you fall asleep, and improves libido.

Fennel E.O. (Foeniculum vulgare)

Fennel essential oil contains phytohormones which have a stimulating effect on the skin and kidneys. It has a diuretic effect and therefore helps eliminate uric acid.

Clary sage E.O. (Salvia sclarea)

Clary sage decreases nervous tension and fatigue. It stimulates blood circulation in the veins.

Other essential oils which you can try include aniseed, cumin, and caraway.

ESSENTIAL OILS
Warning

If a child accidentally absorbs an essential oil, you must immediately call the nearest poison center. Some essential oils can actually cause convulsions if the child ingests excessive quantities thereof.

Alternative medicines

What are the benefits of alternative therapy, such as homeopathy, traditional Chinese medicine, and osteopathy?

Everything that can improve a patient's comfort and well-being is useful. For each of these alternatives, it is useful to consult a specialized professional, doctor, pharmacist, or ostheopath.

Homeopathy: microscopic doses

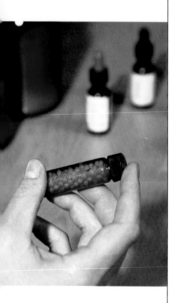

In homeopathy, plants but also products from other natural kingdoms are used: animal and mineral products. There is a very specific way to prepare these drugs. Simultaneously, the raw material is diluted, and the product is made more dynamic. Most of the time, the remedies are soaked onto little sugar lumps or granules, which makes them easier to absorb. The granules must then be dissolved on the tongue. The doses vary greatly. If you self-medicate, it is advisable to use doses of 5C to 9C and to take three granules one to two times a day.

The main homeopathic remedies

Lachesis mutus: When menopause is accompanied by a change in character, intolerance to all tight clothing, hot flashes, migraines, and spontaneous bruising.

Sulfur: When there are simultaneous vascular problems (hot flashes; hemorrhoids), skin problems (acne; rosacea; hives), and joint problems which worsen with heat and improve with the cold.

Sepia officinalis: In women who become sad, short-tempered, cannot tolerate being contradicted, are bloated in the pelvic area, or suffer from internal hot flashes and circulation problems.

Graphites: When menopause is accompanied by chills, weight gain, digestive problems, and hot flashes in the facial area contrasting with a pale complexion.

Thuya occidentalis: for fibroma, warts, and ovarian cysts with pain on the left side.

Numerous remedies can prove useful. We cannot list the m all, but here are some others: *Caulophyllum, Viburnum Opulus, Sabina, Chamomilla, Veratrum Album,* etc. It would undoubtedly be useful to consult a homeopath if you are in doubt or if the above-mentioned products are ineffective. These remedies are the most frequently used, but there are in fact others.

Traditional Chinese medicine

Traditional Chinese medicine includes a number of health practices aimed at preventing and treating diseases, regaining health, and prolonging life. It has multiple facets, including acupuncture (the most well-known in Western society), Chinese plants, massages, but also the art of moving with Tai chi chuan, an increasingly well-known type of gymnastics, and Qi Gong, a breathing technique, where the breath or Qi (pronounced "chee") brings everything in the universe to life..

Osteopathy

Ostheopaths are nothing but gentle. They are attentive to the breaths that maintain life. They know how to accompany the natural movement of your muscles and joints. They can rid you of tensions and help you put more flow into your movements. An ostheopath can help you get back in touch with your body.

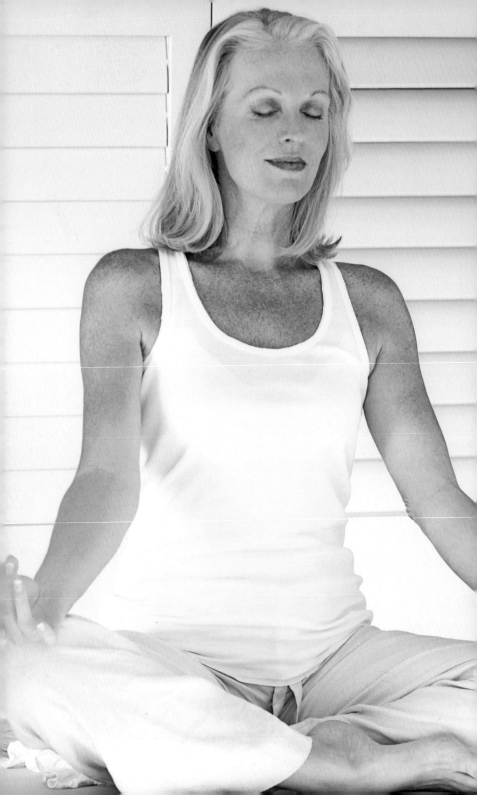

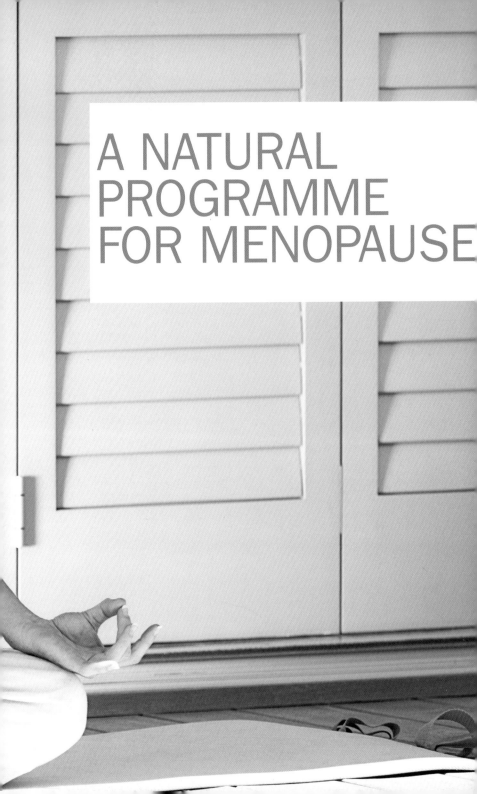

A NATURAL PROGRAMME FOR MENOPAUSE

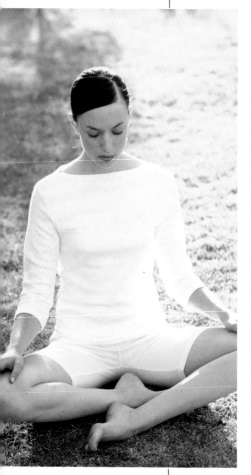

Setting the Record Straight

The age of 50 is the right moment to take stock of one's life. After many years of taking care of others, from spouses and parents to our children, women should take care of themselves! They can begin by having a medical check-up and thereby understand their health much better. First, women should make time to observe themselves and take stock of the following:

•Weight

Aim to be neither too fat nor too thin. It is difficult to battle against thinness because it is most often a product of one's constitution. Avoid being overweight, as it promotes many illnesses. However, the goal must be a reasonable one. It is not about losing too many pounds. Keeping a few curves is also an art of life. Women should not submit themselves to the restrictive images of beauty spread over the pages of women's magazines. Do not hesitate to call upon nutritional experts to help you. Doctors and dieticians have a great deal of knowledge to share.

• Heart rate response

A simple test measures heart rate response. First, take your resting heart rate. Then do a simple exercise that stimulates the heart, for example, 30 rapid lunges. Then take your pulse again and finally a third time after two minutes of rest. Your results are healthy if you return to your resting pulse rate after two minutes and if the pulse taken after the effort of exercise does not exceed 220 pulses per minutes minus your age. For example, for a 50- year-old, you must not exceed 170 beats per minute at exertion. If you surpass this, medical supervision is necessary. You should consideryour heart rate capacity when resuming physical activity and begin with gentle activities at the outset.

• Breasts

Every woman should examine her breasts once a month. No one but you is in a better position to notice changes and to consult a doctor in cases of doubt.

• Joints

Do you experience pains, swollen joints, and back aches that you have hardly ever given a thought?

Stay zen

As our society exposes us to more and more stress, taking anti-stress nutrients and plants may be very useful. However, it is essential to correctly analyze what is happening and attempt to adopt a new way of life. This is where all the relaxation techniques come into play:
•Resting your spirit equals relaxation;
•Resting your body and your spirit equals sleep.
Relaxation enables everybody to become more responsible for his or her health and life. It allows one to rediscover his or her potential and creativity. Relaxation is vital for everyone and it is up to each person to practice relaxation techniques regularly. Although these techniques vary, they have one aspect in common: It is about getting back into touch with one's body and its different functions, particularly breathing, which automatically reduces stress. Relaxation techniques may be used during the course of the day and also at night time in order to fall asleep more easily.

A visit to the doctor

As you approach your 50s, take stock of your health with your GP by having a general check-up and making regular appointments at the gynecologist.

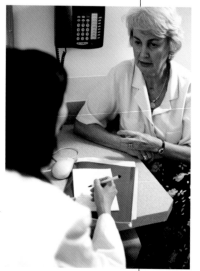

• **The heart:** A few simple tests and a stethoscope examination will allow your doctor to check for a risk of heart disease. Should you be at risk, your doctor will undoubtedly suggest an appointment with a cardiologist. He or she will regularly perform blood tests in order to monitor your overall cholesterol level, your HDL cholesterol (the good cholesterol) level, triglycerides, as well as your blood sugar.

• **Blood vessels:** Your doctor will perform an examination that will enable him or her to check that all the arteries and veins are supple and in good working order. In order to do this, he or she will check your pulse all the way down to your feet and listen to your pulse along your arteries' paths. Your doctor will also examine the state of your veins. Venous dysfunction may give rise to pain or varicose veins in your legs.

• **The bones :** A bone density test will indicate whether your bones are strong or fragile. Depending on the results, your doctor will let you know whether or not you need treatment.

• **The gynecological examination:** Breast cancer is the most common form of cancer in women, usually affecting women between the ages of 50 and 70. It is therefore important to get regular X-rays of your breasts (mammogram) every 2 to 3 years around this age. When your personal risk of breast cancer is higher than that of other women, for example, if someone in your immediate family had breast cancer, it is vital that you are monitored from an early age on.

The screening for cervical cancer entails a pap smear during a gynecological examination. With a pap smear, benign abnormalities can be diagnosed and treated before they progress. If you have had pap smears regularly, and if they never showed any abnormalities, your risk of developing cervical cancer becomes quite low. In this case, you may do a pap smear every 3 years. If you have never had a pap smear before perimenopause, it is important that you have one as soon as possible.

Should you get treatment for your menopause?

After having your medical check-up, the question is whether or not you want to get treatment, and if yes, which kind of treatment would be suitable for you. These decisions need to be thought through. Depending on the intensity of your problems, discomfort, and risk factors, your doctor must explain to you clearly and objectively the different available possibilities. He or she must present all the advantages, disadvantages and possible risks, because if you understand a treatment well, you are more likely to keep to it. Every woman must be able to choose with full knowledge of the facts. The doctor must ensure that the prescribed treatment is indeed the one that suits his patient the best, and the one that his patient is most likely to keep to. He or she must take into account all the patient's expectations. It is the doctor's task to inform the patient and respect her choice, no matter what that may be.

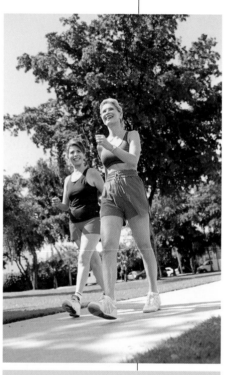

Move, Move, Move!

To combat the risks of osteoporosis and cardiovascular disease, you have to continue moving or start up again if you have not been. Certainly, though, do not exercise in just any old way. Physical activity must be adapted to each individual's potential.

Do not handle your body roughly, or you will find yourself full of aches, pains, and cramps after rashly taking up the sport you played at 18. Go at it slowly and progressively.

Activities you can get started with right away

– walking and swimming
– light exercise, stretching, yoga, or Tai Ji Quan (Chinese exercise)
– aquafit: its greatest advantage comes from the fact that it soothes joints and can be practiced without pain even in the case of overweight women
– biking : start out on flat terrain
– archery
– social dancing
– kayaking

Physical activity gages good health

Getting physical exercise reduces the risk of developing cardiovascular diseases. It also helps you to lose weight, reduce your body fat, and lower your blood pressure.

It decreases your risk of type 2 diabetes and lowers your levels of bad cholesterol.

Women who engage in physical activity for 4 hours a week decrease their risk of breast cancer by 37%. Exercise also enriches your social life.

More intense effort required

After a bit of training in the above-mentioned activities, you can go further:

– running: good quality jogging shoes are essential
– racquet sports such as tennis and badminton. These sports are not advisable for individuals with cardiovascular concerns or high blood pressure.
– cross-country skiing
– golf: not advised for certain back problems or arthrosis
– sailing and rowing

For athletes only

In particular, for those who never gave up their favourite sports:

– horseback riding
– soccer, basketball, volleyball
– wind surfing
– diving
– downhill skiing

How can one get back to exercising at the age of 50?

First of all, one should do a stress test at a cardiologist. If this test shows satisfying results, one can gradually take up exercise again.

First, determine the maximum heart rate (MHR) that you should not exceed during exercise. In theory, this is equal to 220 beats minus your age, but this in fact corresponds to a fit and trained individual. As a beginner, your MHR is 60% of this formula's result. Gradually, you can build it up to 80%.

Therefore, a fit, well-trained, and healthy 50-year-old can run at a speed that allows him or her to reach 170 heartbeats per minute. A beginner's heart rate should not exceed 100 beats per minute. This corresponds to a running speed of approximately 5 miles per hour for the first few weeks of getting back to exercise. Later, you can gradually increase your running speed, but without exceeding 70% of your MHR, i.e., 120 beats per minute.

Do not forget that the somewhat rusty muscles and joints need to be warmed up, for example, with yoga or stretching.

Why not run the half marathon?

Why not bring a little madness into this overly controlled world? There is method in this madness!

A great challenge

Now is the time to do what you never had time to do before. Thanks to the years past and experiences gathered, life has shown you what is good for you. Moreover, what is good for you is also good for the ones close to you. Your good form and mood radiates and brings joy to everybody. Therefore, do yourself some

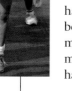

good. For example, set yourself a great challenge by running a half-marathon. The regular training will have wonderful benefits for you, day after day: an increasingly good physical condition, a permanent good mood, patience when confronting hardships, and joy. Who knows, maybe you can beat 88-year old Fenya Crown, who ran the Rome marathon on 25 March 2001 in 7 hours, 29 minutes, and 3 seconds? But rather start with a half-marathon!

Gradual training

Perseverance is a personal trait is necessary from the start. Through perseverance, you will go far, or even better, get a friend to face the challenge with you.

Every training cycle is completed over 4 weeks, or if you do no have enough time, four times 9 days. You will need to train three times every 7- to 9-day cycle, or every 2 to 3 days.

Week 1

Workout No. 1: 30 minutes alternating running and walking, ending with 10 min. of running

Workout No. 2: 45 minutes alternating running and walking, ending with 15 min. of running

Workout No. 3: 90 minutes of running, walking, and biking.

Week 2

Workout No. 1: 45 minutes alternating running and walking, ending with 15 min. of running

Workout No. 2: 60 minutes alternating running and walking, ending with 20 min. of running

Workout No. 3: total of two hours: 30 min. of walking, followed by alternating running and walking.

Week 3

Workout No. 1: 45 minutes alternating running and walking, ending with 15 min. of running

Workout No. 2: 60 minutes alternating running and walking, ending with 20 min. of running

Workout No. 3: total of two hours: 30 min. of walking, followed by alternating running, walking, and biking.

Week 4: Recovery Program

Workout No. 1: biking or walking for one hour

Workout No. 2: 30 minutes alternating 45 seconds of running with 15 seconds of walking

Workout No. 3: biking or walking for 60 to 75 minutes.

Then begin a new cycle of four weeks, gradually increasing the length of time spent running.

Before facing up to this challenge, have your doctor perform a thorough check-up on you in order to make sure that everything is in working order and that you are only a little rusty! While you are running, check your heart rate and adjust your running speed.

Living Well Means Eating Well

A healthy, varied diet delights the eyes, the heart, and the body.

Every day, respect the following balance

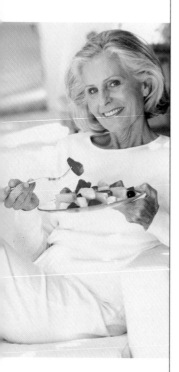

• **15 % proteins.** The ideal is to consume half of your protein from animal sources (preferably white meat, fish, eggs, and dairy products) and the other half from plant sources (grains, especially whole, and legumes, such as soy). For vegetarians, plant proteins must come from two different sources. One source must be a grain and the other, a legume. For example, the combination of rice and lentils is a good one because it provides the essential amino acids. Only two plant sources provide all the amino acids on their own: soy and quinoa.

• **30 to 35% lipids (fat).** It is certain that the quality of the fats we eat influences the quality of our arteries, our hormones, and our mood. Good fats can be distinguished from the bad ones by the fatty acids they contain. Good fats are the unsaturated fatty acids, and the less good, indeed bad ones, are the saturated fatty acids found in butter, dairy products, cheese, cold cuts, and certain meats such as lamb. Consume these bad fats in moderation because they increase the risk of heart disease and probably even certain cancers. Unsaturated fatty acids are found in vegetable oils. The most attractive for health are those that contain the essential fatty acids. The best oils are olive oil and canola oil. Canola contains the two essential fatty acids, linoleic acid and alphalinoleic acid, in ideal proportions. As for olive oil, it contains oleic acid, which protects fats from oxidation. Dried oleaginous plants (nuts of all kinds) are a good source of high-quality fats.

• **50 to 55 % de carbohydrates.** Be careful, because there are good and bad in this grouping as well. Foods with a high glycemic index make blood sugar levels increase very quickly (sugar, soft drinks, white rice, white flour, chips, and French fries). Carbohydrates also hide in baked goods, dairy products, popcorn, corn flakes, most breakfast cereals, instant rice, fast food buns, etc. Avoid simple sugars as much as possible and get into the habit of using low glycemic index sugars, which are distributed throughout the body very slowly. They maintain blood sugar levels at a constant rate and are true fat burners. They are the best fuels for the brain and muscles by allowing them to function well both at rest and for the duration. The following are some low glycemic index foods: whole wheat bread, whole rye bread, whole wheat pasta, brown rice, almost all vegetables and fresh fruit, soy, lentils, and plain, unsweetened yogurt.

Eat three square meals per day:
– Breakfast: 25% of the day's calories (rich in proteins)
– Lunch: 40% (rich in proteins)
– Dinner: 35% (rich in complex carbohydrates)

Vitamins must accompany the three macronutrients so that the body can properly make use of them. Obtain the necessary vitamins by eating three fresh fruit, one serving of raw vegetables, and a portion of salad every day.

Choosing well means eating well

Choose the foods containing compounds which protect your health..

- Unsaturated omega-3 fatty acids: oily fish, camelina or rapeseed oil, lettuce, soy, and all types of nuts.
- Monounsaturated fats: olive oil, olives, almonds, foie gras, confit of goose, and avocado.
- Slow-release sugars: wholegrain levain bread, wholegrain bread, whole grains, legumes, and starches.
- Foods rich in arginine, ornithine, and polyamines: oil-producing plants, crucifers, legumes, legume sprouts, soy and soy products, and green tea.
- Foods rich in sulfur containing amino acids: seafood, fish, eggs, asparagus, leeks, crucifers, onion, and garlic.
- Sulfates: certain bottled mineral waters.
- Potassium: dried fruits, oil-producing plants, fruits (bananas), legumes, soy, and whole grains.
- Calcium: certain bottled mineral waters, calcium-enriched soy milk, gruyère, emmenthal, parmesan, yogurt, crucifers, beets, whole sardines, almonds, and walnuts.
- Magnesium: most calcium-rich mineral water, soy, oil-producing plants, whole grains, legumes, green vegetables, fish, and periwinkles.
- Zinc: shellfish, fish, meat, liver, eggs, and ginger.
- Selenium: Brazil nuts, fish, seafood, meat, liver, grains, red pepper, boletus mushrooms, and garlic (depending

Eating with Pleasure

The ideal is to meet with friends in a lovely setting. Take the time to eat slowly. Put aside the cares of the day, and eat sitting down.

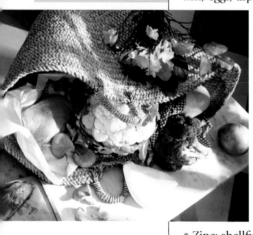

Eating well means avoiding foods that accelerate aging

- Saturated fats: cold cuts, pork, butter, peanut oil, fried foods.
- Trans fats: hydrogenated oils and margarines, "fast food" fried foods.
- Excess simple sugars: candy, jam, sweetened drinks, white bread.
- Excess sodium (salt), iron, or copper.
- Heavy metals and nitrates
- Hidden fats, sugar, and salt.

Despite the fact that there is so little time left after working and taking care of the house and the children... find your way back to your kitchen. It is better to eat fresh food, cooked by your own hands, than prepared foods that are rich in sugar, fat, and salt, and in artificial sweeteners and colourings.

on the richness of the soil).

• Silica: whole grains and mineral water.

• Vitamins B1, B3, B6, B9, B12, C, and E: yeast such as malt, whole grains, and legumes.

• Beta-carotene: red fruit and vegetables, carrots, and blueberries.

• Lycopene: tomato sauce, cooked tomato, papaya, pink grapefruit, and watermelon.

• Live cultures (Bifidus, Lactobacillus, etc.): yogurt and sauerkraut.

During menopause, one should particularly choose foods which are rich in phytoestrogens of which soy is an essential food.

Magnesium deficiency is a common problem

Modern lifestyles tend to cause stress, which makes it even more necessary to get sufficient magnesium. This mineral is found in some foods which are oh so good, oh so smooth but oh so high in calories: chocolate, dried fruit, and bananas. However, magnesium can also be found in whole grains, seafood, oily fish, vegetables, and whole-grain bread. Adults need 300 to 700mg of magnesium per day, depending on their lifestyle. The more stressful their lifestyle is, the more magnesium they need. In the United States, at least 68% of the population presents a magnesium deficiency. This deficiency manifests itself in several little ways, ranging from a tingling sensation in the extremities to depression. There is no risk of overdosing in magnesium. If you consume too much magnesium in the form of a supplement, it will be naturally excreted by your body but may sometimes cause diarrhea.

Taking vitamin and mineral supplements
means protecting yourself!

"Vitamin and mineral supplements are not useful if one does have a balanced and varied diet." Today, this statement is being re-examined by a number of experts.

Less calories means less vitamins and minerals

Modern lifestyles cause women to have to run about, from the office to their home, to the apartment where the youngest in the family has just moved in, to the parents who need help, and the best friend who is feeling terribly depressed. How can they still do their grocery shopping at the local organic store, remember to soak the chickpeas before cooking them, and cook a healthy and flavorsome meal containing plenty of vitamins and minerals? Moreover, life has changed. We are increasingly stressed, but we spent much less physical energy than before. This is why our calorie requirements have also decreased. In order to get sufficient quantities of vitamins, minerals, and trace elements, we would surely have to increase the amount of calories we take in every day. This puts us at risk of gaining weight, which is not something that we want.

Dietary supplements can therefore help us. They are available at the pharmacy, drugstore, and in diet stores. However, be careful, as not all supplements are suited for everyone.

Do you lack vitamins? Below is a list of what you could be risking.

Situation	Biochemical consequences	Metabolic consequences	Menopausal Women at risk
Deficiency in antioxidants (vitamins C and E, selenium, and zinc)	Decreased protection against free radicals	- Weaker immune system - Risk of heart attack or stroke - Risk of cataracts and age-related macular degeneration - Increased vulnerability to infection	- Passive and active smokers - Women living in cities (pollution) - Asthmatics - Women who love the sun - Women consuming only small amounts of fruit and vegetables
Deficiency in vitamins B1, B2, B3, B5, B6, C, and magnesium	Lowered activity of neurotransmitters involved in memory and alertness	- Risk of cognitive problems - Risk of Alzheimer's disease and Parkinson's disease - Risk of colo-rectal cancer	- Women who consume large amounts of sweet foods - Elderly persons
Deficiency in vitamins B6, B9, and B12	Increase in homocysteine (a toxic product of the breaking down of protein)	- Risk of depression - Risk of heart attack or stroke	All women
Vitamin D deficiency	- Bone loss or bone changes - Lowered protection against cancer initiation - Risk of osteoporosis - Risk of skin, breast, and colon cancer		Women living in cities, winter

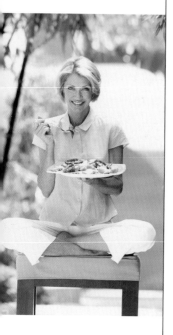

Stock up on antioxidants means protecting yourself !

Antioxidants play an essential role in the fight against ageing and in the prevention of certain diseases. They work in synergy in our body.

Carotenoids: beta-carotene (provitamin A), lycopene

High levels of beta-carotene in the blood are linked to a decreased risk of developing some cancers. Carotenoids also lower the risk of cataracts and retinal macular degeneration.

They are found in carrots, cauliflower, red spices (red chili; paprika), and yellow fruit (apricots, mangos, cantaloupes, and watermelons). Large quantities of lycopene are found in tomatoes, broccoli, and spinach. Beta-carotene is contained in some dietary supplements.

Vitamin C

There is some controversy about vitamin C requirements. Some consider that 10 to 100mg per day are sufficient, whereas others suggest four to ten times higher doses. Active and passive smokers, women who take the contraceptive pill, asthmatics, diabetics, and persons suffering from chronic diseases need at least 500mg per day.

Vitamin C is found in fresh fruit such as kiwi, acerola, rose hip, and citrus fruit. Vitamin C supplements can be taken by anyone except those suffering from hemochromatosis and kidney dysfunction.

Vitamin E

Vitamin E is a very powerful antioxidant, which protects the cell from the attack of free radicals.

It is found in wheat germ oil, almonds, and hazelnuts. It is difficult to determine the required amounts. Vitamin E deficiency is a common problem, and the amount needed increases in excessively strict slimming diets and certain diseases. If you need supplements, choose those containing natural vitamin E. There is no risk of overdosing on vitamin E, but persons who are scheduled to undergo an operation, who suffer from a disease affecting their eyesight known as *retinitis pigmentosa,* as well as hemophiliacs should be cautious.

Selenium

This powerful antioxidant slows down cell ageing and also acts as a detoxifying agent. By binding itself to heavy metals, it enables the body to excrete them in the urine. It also has an effect on blood fluidity.

It is found, above all, in fish, seafood, eggs, and meat. Certain plant products (grains in particular) may also contain some selenium, depending on the soil's richness. Selenium is contained in many dietary supplements.

Zinc

Zinc plays a role in the regulation of genes, insulin, the immune defense, and eyesight. Moreover, zinc also displays antioxidant properties in the body.

It is found in, above all, meat, fish, and seafood. Over 70% of people in the United States are consuming less than the recommended allowance of zinc. Zinc is enclosed in some multivitamin preparations, which are sold in pharmacies.

Selenium and Cancer

Selenium deficiency can promote certain cancers (prostate, breast, colon, and liver). In the United States, a double-blind, placebo-controlled study of 1,312 individuals showed that, in the group that took a selenium supplement (200 µg/day), total cancer mortality was cut in half.

More solid bones

In order to prevent osteoporosis, one needs calcium. An intake of 1.2 to 1.5g of calcium per day would be ideal. However, this is not sufficient.

Calcium is the main building block of bones, and 99% of calcium is stored in the bones. Although it is vital to supply the body with sufficient amounts of this mineral, this is not enough to ensure strong bones. In fact, the absorption, retention, and binding of calcium to the bones strongly depend on numerous conditions: physical activity, the acid-base balance, but also the presence of vitamin D.

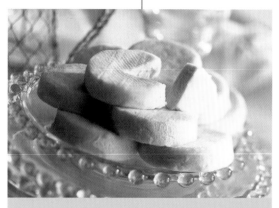

Dairy products in moderation

Cheese is not recommendable for women who gain weight easily, as it often contains high levels of fat. However, goat's cheese and sheep's cheese contain less fat than cow's milk cheeses. Note that several large studies, one of which was conducted on 80,000 women, did not demonstrate that the consumption of dairy products prevents osteoporotic fractures.

Where is calcium found?

Milk and milk products, of course, contain calcium. However, those who do not like dairy products may find enough calcium in vegetables, dried fruit, and calcium-rich mineral water. Calcium can also be taken as a supplement in the form of tablets, vials, or powder. It is often necessary to associate it with vitamin D3. Ask your doctor for advice, as persons suffering from certain diseases, such as hypercalcemia and severe kidney dysfunction, should not take calcium.

Is vitamin D essential for bone strength?

Our body gets this vitamin especially through sun exposure. This is quite problematic in winter, even if you expose your face and arms to the sun, as the sun's rays have weaker effects in winter. The vitamin D levels in the blood are lowered, which can cause deficiencies with heavy consequences, especially in persons older than 50. Small amounts of vitamin D are also found in foods such as oily fish, egg yolk, liver, and dairy products. Vitamin D3 supplements are necessary during winter and fall.

Watch your acid-base balance

When the body is too acidic, due to a diet too high in animal proteins and grains, it regains its balance by taking calcium from the bones where this mineral is stored. One essential element in the acid-base regulation is potassium, which is contained in fruit and vegetables or may be purchased in the form of supplements. It allows the body to strengthen bones, while slowing down the depletion of calcium.

Exercise, of course!

Although populations in developing countries consume little calcium, they do not have an osteoporosis problem, probably because they are more active than we are. All exercise is good for bones, except swimming, because not enough pressure is exerted on the bones during this activity.

Today, there are several effective treatments for fighting osteoporosis (*see page 54*).

Calcium-rich foods (mg/100g)

Plain yogurt	140–170
Hard cheese:	
emmental	1 000
Goat's cheese	140
Fresh sardines	290
Almonds	250
Mung beans	255
Fresh parsley	200
Shrimps	200
Watercress	160
Dried figs	160
Green olives	100
Cooked spinach	256
Chicory	100
Cooked broccoli	100
Egg yolk	140
Cooked white beans	60
Cooked red beans	112

Calcium-rich beverages (mg/L)

Milk	1 200
Certain mineral waters	545

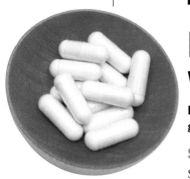

Treating Hot Flashes with Soy

Hot flashes are the sign of a deficiency of estrogens. Soy extracts can help to treat them.

Soy: Natural or extract form

Soy can be used as a food or also as a dietary supplement in the form of gel capsules that contain a standardized soyisoflavone extract. Studies show that consuming 35 to 80 mg of soy isoflavones per day results in a reduction in the frequency and intensity of hot flashes. Start with 35 mg per day. You should wait 20 days before judging the dosage's effectiveness. However, it is possible to increase the dosage without problems (multiply by two or four), and spread them out through the day. For example, to avoid night sweats, take two gel capsules before bedtime.

Choosing a food supplement rich in phytoestrogens

The dosage required to supply sufficient phytohormones must be greater than 35 mg of isoflavones per day. In Europe currently, diet provides only 5 mg. It might be worthwhile then for European women to take soyextract based dietary supplements. These products are more and more in demand, and their numbers are constantly growing. Most contain soy extracts, to which ingredients such as wild yam extract, magnesium, and anti-oxidants are sometimes added.

The most important thing to be aware of is the quantity of isoflavones available in each gel capsule. Indeed, soy and soy extracts contain highly varying quantities of isoflavones according to the type of soy, the location it was grown, and the time it was harvested. The ideal daily isoflavone dosage is 35 to 90 mg. Taking more is hazardous. Turn to products that have been the subject of serious clinical studies published in medical journals. It is best to follow the advice of health care professional.

Where is research headed?

Biochemists are trying to understand which are the active molecules in soy. They extracted genisteine, diadzeine, and glyciteine, and then synthesized a new molecule using daidzeine: ipriflavone. This molecule has proven to be particularly useful in treating osteoporosis. Several studies have demonstrated its effectiveness so well that today the substance is proposed in Italy, Japan, and Hungary. Unfortunately, we do not have the necessary hindsight to be to able to affirm that the molecule has no side effects. Research on this subject is ongoing.

Phytoestrogens in salad

Phytoestrogens are found in more than 600 plants, not all of which are edible. We can only use approximately 20 of these plants.

The main dietary sources of phytoestrogens are lis ted below:

• **Sources of isoflavones:** soy beans, chickpeas, lentils, onions, apples, green beans, grapes, olive oil, red wine, citrus fruit, green tea, and black tea. The best sources of isoflavones are soy beans.

• **Sources of lignans:** whole-wheat grains, oily grains (flaxseed; olive; sunflower), flageolets, lentils, cherries, apples, pears, grapefruit, garlic, green tea, and black tea. The best source of lignans is flaxseed.

• **Sources of coumestans:** soy and alfalfa sprouts, which are used in some cooking recipes.

Small dinner menu

Dandelion and olive salad, followed by cream of chickpea and fennel soup.

This small meal contains 450kcal and exhibits a good balance between macronutrients and micronutrients. Fennel, chickpeas, soy, and garlic are rich in phytohormones.

Dandelion and olive salad

7 to 9oz of dandelion
Two slices of stale bread
24 black olives
1 ½ oz of parmesan
One clove of garlic
One tablespoon of balsamic vinegar
Three tablespoons of olive oil
Salt; pepper

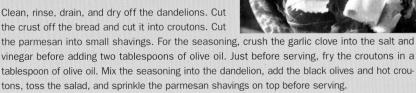

Clean, rinse, drain, and dry off the dandelions. Cut the crust off the bread and cut it into croutons. Cut the parmesan into small shavings. For the seasoning, crush the garlic clove into the salt and vinegar before adding two tablespoons of olive oil. Just before serving, fry the croutons in a tablespoon of olive oil. Mix the seasoning into the dandelion, add the black olives and hot croutons, toss the salad, and sprinkle the parmesan shavings on top before serving.

Cream of chickpea and fennel soup

18oz fennel bulbs
3 ½ oz of chickpeas
Two cloves of garlic
Just over half a pint of soy milk
Salt; pepper
Chopped fennel leaves

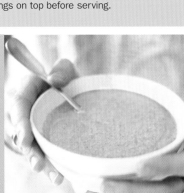

The day before, leave the chickpeas to soak in water. Cook them using the basic recipe. While they are cooking, wash the fennel, cut off the hard, bruised, and stringy parts. Keep the green leaves, cut them into strips, and boil them with the garlic, salt, and pepper in one and a half pints of water for 20 minutes. Check the pot every now and then. Take the two pots and put the contents into a blender until you are left with a very smooth puree. Put the puree back into the pot with the soy milk, and sprinkle the remaining chopped fennel over it.

Treat hot flashes with other plants

Several plants may complement the effect of soy on hot flashes.

Black cohosh
(Cimicifuga racemosa; Actea racemosa)

Originally from North America, black cohosh was used by Native Americans in order to treat menstrual problems. It was recently rediscovered and studied in a German research unit in the 1990s. The dried root of this plant is used as a brew or a mother tincture, which is prepared in pharmacies. Black cohosh acts on the serotonin receptors, but it appears not to have an estrogenic effect. The plant is essentially used for gynecological and rheumatic problems, as it relieves painful periods. It relieves problems related to excess progesterone and menopause, such as fatigue, sadness, and hot flashes. The plant also has a sedative effect.
Brew: Drink one cup two times a day.
Mother tincture: Take 50 drops three times a day.

Oats (Avena sativa)

Originally from Northern Europe, oats are cultivated everywhere and have already been used for the nervous system for many years. This plant remedies depression, improves libido, and is fortifying.
In our diet, it is used in the form of oat flakes. It can also be bought in the form of capsules, teas, mother tinctures, and liquid extracts.

Common sage (Salvia officinalis)

For many years, sage has been considered to be a cure-all, which gives us an explanation for its Latin name, as Salvia means "save". Sage has many effects, such as anti-septic, tonic, and digestive activities. It is also a hormone stimulant, regulates the menstrual cycle, and displays estrogen-like effects. Moreover, sage regulates perspiration, which makes it a very good remedy for hot flashes. The leaves of this plant are used fresh or dried, and can also be taken as capsules, teas, or as a mother tincture. It is contra-indicated during pregnancy and in hormone-dependant cancer patients.

Hop (Humulus lupulus)

Originally from Europe and Asia, hop is mainly used for brewing beer. However, the plant also has medicinal properties.
Hop is a tonic for the digestive system and exhibits seda-tive and estrogen-like effects. It reduces nervousness. The female flowers (or strobiles) are used in teas, as capsules, or as mother tinctures. It is best to avoid hop if one suffers from depression.

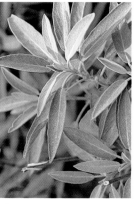

Sage

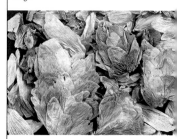

Hop

Many other plants have estrogen-like effects. These include licorice, pussy willow, scarlet pimpernel, flaxseed, marigold, grapefruit juice, dong quai, and alfalfa

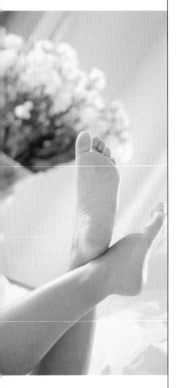

Recover light legs

During menopause, numerous American women complain of leg problems. According to the doctors, this may be accounted for by a lack of exercise, smoking, desk-bound jobs, and excess weight. In the following you can read what you should do about it.

The veins in the lower limbs must ensure that the blood flows back to the heart by making light work of gravity. In order to do this, the entire leg has to get involved: When the muscles contract, they push the blood upwards with the help of the vein wall's flexibility. However, all this effort would be in vain were it not for the valves spaced out all along the walls, preventing the blood to flow back towards the feet. Tingling, prickling, night cramps, and heavy legs are indicative of the dysfunctioning of one of the three components. While blood stagnates in the veins, these become wider and turn into varicose veins.

However, this is not deadly. Doctors advise those who are at risk or already suffer from heavy legs to walk, swim, and cycle, which reduces pressure on the veins. If you have a desk-bound job, flex your knees and ankles frequently, get up, and walk. At the end of the day, lift your legs so that they are approximately one foot higher than your heart.

Stimulate your blood flow

Ideally, your diet should provide you with three portions of fruit and three to six portions of vegetables per day. Fruit and vegetables contain flavanoids which fight inflammation, make the blood more fluid, stimulate venous contractions, reinforce the vein walls, and protect against the harmful actions of oxygen breakdown products. You can also find them in wine (do not drink more than one glass a day), tea, herbal tea, grape juice, and even chocolate! If you require a more radical solution, turn to plants. They are extraordinary little factories which synthesize flavanoids, saponosids, and other antioxidants that your legs need (read insert). Lastly, for seasoning your vegetables, use oils rich in omega-3 fatty acids, such as rapeseed, nut, and soy oil. They will render your blood more fluid and give you the final push necessary *for the all-important venous return.*

Artery-Friendly Plants

Phytotherapy effectively relieves blood circulation problems such as heavy legs, varicose veins, and hemorrhoids. The following can be found in pharmacies and health food stores in either gel capsules or ready-to-use liquid extracts:

Witchhazel is a powerful vascoconstrictor and cicatrisation agent. Both the bark and leaves are used.

Ginkgo biloba (leaf) acts on micro - circulation and peripheral circulation. It protects the brain against cerebral vascular accidents (stroke).

Horse-chestnut (bark) reduces capillary permeability and is an anti- edemic.

Red vine (leaf and fruit) is an ideal tonic for veins and reduces capillary permeability.

Ruscus is a vein tonic and diuretic. It also improves capillary resistance.

Sweet clover improves blood consistency and reduces inflammation.

..And for the bladder

The mucous membrane of the bladder becomes very sensitive as hormones diminish. There may be pain when urinating, frequent urges, or an inability to empty the bladder, which are not caused by infection, but by inflammation. In this case, several plants are helpful:

Bearberry is an antiseptic and astringent;

Juniper is a diuretic, antiseptic, and analgesic;

Propolisresin is a natural anti-inflammatory ;

Rosemary is an antiseptic.

Be in a good mood again naturally

During menopause, women are often plagued by sleeping problems. Sleep disturbances often worsen the stress and anxiety that this period of life brings along. However, there are solutions.

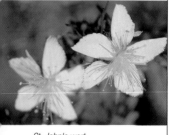

St. John's wort

The usual treatment for stress, insomnia, and anxiety generally entails drugs known as benzodiazepines, which are antidepressant drugs. These drugs all have potential side effects and can also cause patients to become dependent on them. Before taking antidepressants, ask your doctor or pharmacist for advice on herbal remedies and dietary supplements. Herebelow, we have listed some useful plants, one of which your doctor might suggest to you.

Natural treatments for sleep and mood disturbances

Substance	Indications principales	Posologie
Hawthorn	Stress; anxiety	Capsules: 1 to 2g per day, divided into 3 doses
Black horehound	Stress; anxiety	Capsules: 1 to 2g per day, divided into 3 doses
Passion flower	Insomnia	Capsules: 1 to 2g per day, divided into 3 doses
Valerian	Insomnia; tobacco detoxification	Capsules: 1 to 2g per day, divided into 3 doses
St. John's wort	Light to moderate depression	Capsules: 600mg to 1g per day, divided into 3 doses
Ginseng	Insomnia related to nervous fatigue	Capsules: 1 to 2g per day, divided into 3 doses
Magnesium	Chronic stress (with irritable bowel syndrome) anxiety due to premenstrual syndrome	500 mg per day
Folic acid (EPA; DHA)	irritability	500 to 5 000 mg per day (always taken with vitamin B12)
Nicotinamide	Insomnia with anxiety, or irritability, mood swings and light bipolar depression	500 to 1 500 mg in the evening
Cobalamin	Insomnia with sleep-wake rhythm disturbances or uncontrolled movement	1 000 mg par jour per day (one vial in water just after dinner)
Fish oils (EPA, DHA)	agressiveness, chronic stress	Capsules: 3 per day, divided into 3 doses

NB.: This table is based on research data. The products, dosage, and possible combinations must be adjusted to your case, particularly as there are contra-indications and possible interactions with other drugs. It is essential that you consult your doctor or pharmacist before consuming the abovementioned products. All these products are available in pharmacies.

St. John's wort: a natural and safe alternative to antidepressants

On 3 August 1996, the prestigious *British Medical Journal* published a study conducted by a group of researchers on a depression treatment. The researchers summed up the results of 23 studies in which patients were given an herbal remedy, whereas the others were given a placebo. Their conclusion was that the herbal remedy was significantly more effective than the placebo on the symptoms of light to moderate depression. St. John's wort has recently made a dramatic entrance in the world of medicine. Since 1996, St. John's wort has been tested in many other clinical trials. Not only does this plant improve light to moderate depression but it also appears to be just as effective as conventional treatments, with only minor side effects.

However, **St. John's wort does not treat severe depression.** Only a doctor can judge the severity of the depression and the possible benefit of St. John's wort.

This plant may cause some side effects, particularly in the digestive system. It is contra-indicated during pregnancy and breastfeeding. Also be careful of its interaction with certain drugs such as oral contraceptives, anti-vitamin K agents, theophylline, antiretrovirals, and certain immunosuppressants.

Prior to their recent marketing authorization, Arkopharma capsules containing dry St. John's wort extract, the powder form of St. John's wort, were prohibited in France. Today, the capsules provide a part of the 1.2 million patients and their doctors with a natural, confirmed, and alternative therapy. In the United States, St. John's wort is a widely used ad popular supplement sold as capsules, tablets, teas, and liquid extracts.

Lithium: an antidepressant trace element

Thanks to its neurosedative effects, lithium plays a vital role in treating symptoms of nervousness with sleep disturbances, irritability, and anxiety. It also relieves headache in menopausal women. High doses of lithium are used in the psychiatric treatment of manic-depressive disorders.

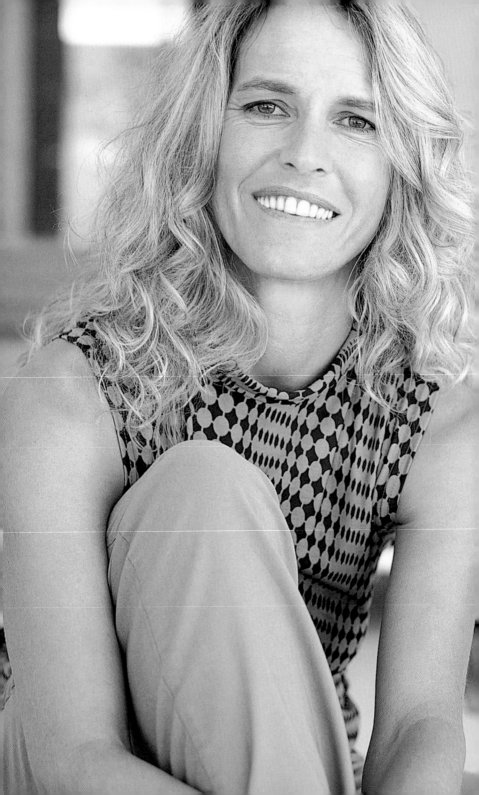

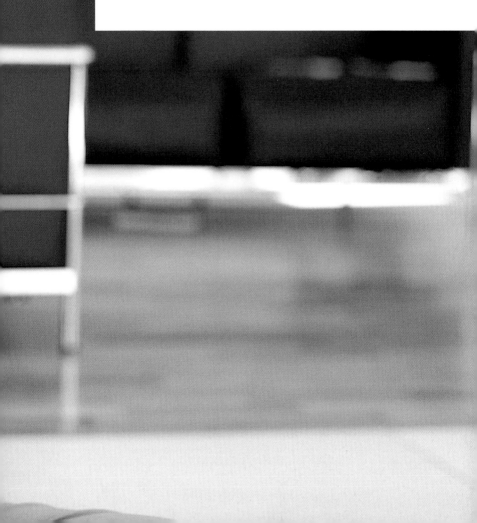

CONCLUSION

A Health Programme for all Women

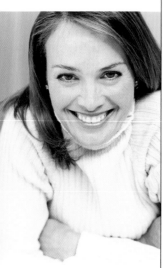

This period of hormonal imbalance in a woman's life is truly unpleasant. The calendar cannot be trusted. Menstrual periods show up too early or too late. At certain times, there is almost no flow; at others, the flow is almost a hemorrhage. Hot flashes begin to make themselves known. A little bit of anxiety casts a shadow over everyday life. If you are not careful, tension and insomnia settle in. Eventually, these difficulties cloud the entire picture of your life. It is high time to discover a new art of living, and to put into practice all of your newly-acquired knowledge to really savour the tenderness of life.

Rediscover the art of eating well

Invite the sun to your table with fruit and vegetables of all colours. Enrich your table with recipes that are rich in fibre; the whole grains will be there, in perfect harmony with the legumes. The meat will stay discreet, along with the butter and fresh cream. The fish will supply you regularly with its fatty acids. Delicious, healthy olive and canola oils will flavour the salads and raw vegetables. Soy in all its forms will be there to help regulate your capricious hormonal activity a little..

Learn to move again

The days pass from one to the next and all look alike, always running after the clock between the offic e, the house, and the household chores. You are overcome with exhaustion, and once the evening arrives, you collapse in front of a television that hypnotizes you, but does not let you truly rest. It is time to change all that. Begin by cutting back one or two nights of television per week. Rediscover yourself with your partner or best friend in a relaxing activity: some aquafit or a stroll along the canal or in the nearest forest. This first bit of relaxation will give you the urge to go even further and to begin (or begin again) an athletic activity that will bring flexibility to your joints, strength to your muscles, and calming relief to your spirit..

Relieve your stress

Numerous techniques exist to help you: yoga and breathing techniques, sophrology, *Qi Gong*, the Vittoz method, and autogenic training are but a few. Plants, vitamin supplements, minerals, and trace elements will also help you. If this is not enough, it is never too late to begin working with a psychologist to understand better why so much of what you experience is stressful.

Tame your hormones

A few plants will help stabilize your cycles and decrease hot flashes: evening primrose, sage, black cohosh, and hops. Of course, do not forget soy -i s o flavone dietary supplements, which decrease the frequency and intensity of hot flashes. Consider ginger, too: it restores normal sleep patterns, puts an end to palpitations, and improves libido.

If you cannot make it alone, consult your doctor.

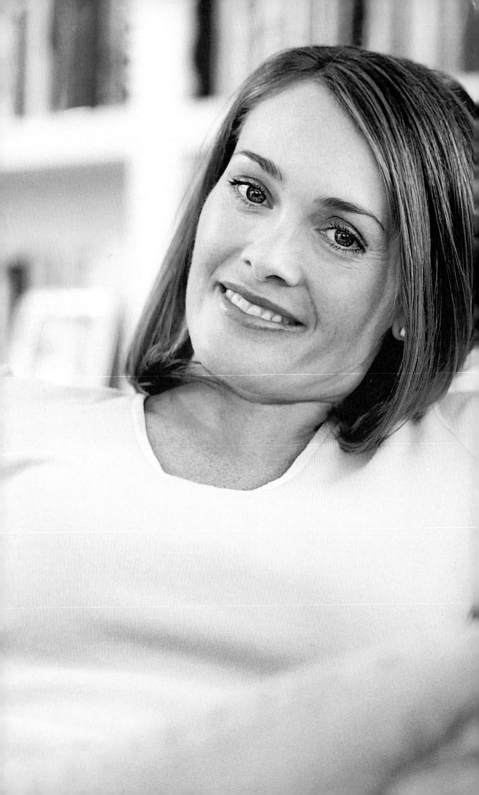

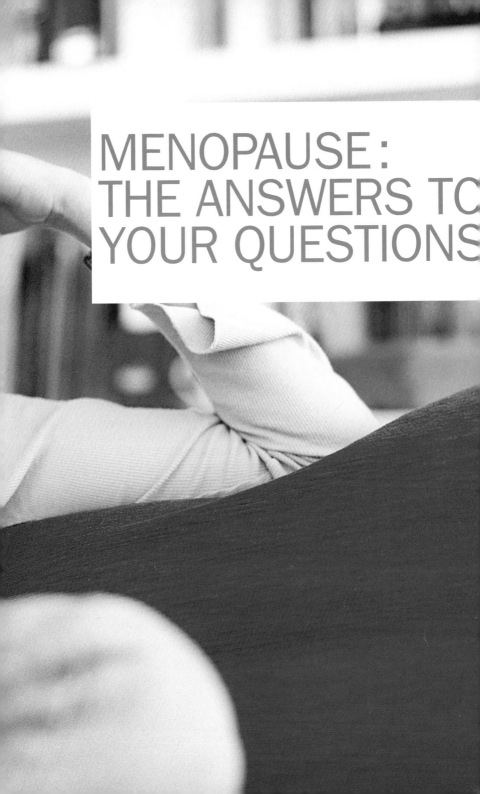

MENOPAUSE: THE ANSWERS TO YOUR QUESTIONS

MENOPAUSE:
THE ANSWERS TO YOUR QUESTIONS

Are hot flashes frequent, and how long do they last?

Hot flashes at menopause bother around 70% of women who follow Western lifestyle. Among Asian women, they affect only 30% of menopausal women. On average, they last for three years, then fade away little by little to disappear after five to eight years in total. However, they may bother some women for more than 10 years.

Do hot flashes occur at a particular time of day?

For many women, the first hot flashes appear at night and then during the day. Sometimes, the opposite is true. But for all women, certain factors trigger them: stress, nervousness, fatigue, and the consumption of alcohol, coffee, spices, or tobacco.

Can eating soy prevent cancers ?

Studies indicate that individuals who consume many foods containing phytoestrogens—including soy— have less risk of developing breast, endometrial, or colon cancer. However, other studies have not reached the same conclusions. For the time being, soy's role in cancer prevention is theoretical.

What is certain is that the lifestyle of Asian women reduces their risk of developing breast or endometrial cancer. The hypothesis that this reduction is linked to the consumption of phytoestrogens is probable. Nevertheless, other factors certainly come into play.

Do phytoestrogens cause cancer ?

Phytoestrogens contained in food do not increase the risk of developing cancer. On the other hand, high doses of phytoestrogens taken in the form of food supplements have not been proven harmless. As a precaution, women with hormone-dependent cancers are advised not to consume phytoestrogens.

Can phytoestrogens prevent cardiovascular disease?

The daily ingestion of soy proteins instead of animal proteins leads to a reduction of total cholesterol and of bad cholesterol (LDL). Soy also decreases triglyceride levels. Isoflavones taken alone, however, do not provide as effective action. In the United States, it is acknowledged that daily consumption of 25 grams of soy protein, in conjunction with a low-fat diet, reduces the risk of coronary disease.

Is it necessary to consume phytoestrogens throughout one's lifetime and more specifically when there is a risk of breast cancer ?

The consumption of soy, the food richest in phytoestrogens, is advised for everyone, and particularly women at risk of breast cancer. However, for the time being, the consumption of dietary supplements high in phytoestrogens cannot be included in this general advice. There have not been numerous enough scientific studies conducted to prove their effectiveness and to assess potential risk.

Can you replace cow's milk with soy milk?

Soy milk has 35 calories (kcal) per 100 g serving; partially-skimmed cow's milk has 48. If you suffer from cow's milk protein intolerance, then soy milk is a good choice. It is also a good choice if you wish to lower high cholesterol leve l s. Make sure to choose soy milk enriched with calcium, for it naturally contains very little (21 mg per 100 g, as opposed to 118 mg per 100 g in cow's milk).

GLOSSARY

FATTY ACIDS: main element in fats.

ESSENTIAL FATTY ACID: fatty acid that the body cannot produce though it is vital to us.

PLATELET AGGREGATION: phenomenon where platelets stick together, for example, in order to stop bleeding. Hyperaggregation of platelets increases the risk of blood clots.

ANEMIA: decreased quantity of hemoglobin in the blood. This decrease is almost always proportionate to the decrease of red blood cells.

ANGINA PECTORIS: (syn. angor) pain which generally occurs in the thorax, is often constrictive, and may be linked to a heart attack.

ANTIOXIDANT: substance which protects the body against free radicals (substances produced in the body during oxidation).

ATHEROMA: fat and oxidated cholesterol deposits in arteries, with a thickening of the vessel wall and the formation of fibrous tissue.

ATHEROSCLEROSIS: hardening and thickening of arteries due to the accumulation of oxidated fats, such as LDL cholesterol particles. The clustering of particles leads to the formation of atherosclerotic plaques which reduce the lumen of the artery, thereby slowing down blood flow.

CANDIDA ALBICANS: microscopic fungus causing yeast infections (oral thrush or vaginal infections).

YELLOW BODY: temporary gland which is formed in the ovarian follicles after the release of an ovum during ovulation.

ADRENAL CORTEX: area around the adrenal gland, which itself is found above the kidneys.

BREW: way of preparing plants by boiling dried or fresh plants in water for approximately 10 to 20 minutes.

ENDOMETRIUM: mucous membrane lining the internal wall of the uterus.

UTERINE FIBROMA: benign tumor which develops at the expense of the muscular tissue of the uterus.

OVARIAN FOLLICLE: small anatomical formation found in the ovaries which resembles a small bag and contains an oocyte.

CARBOHYDRATES: also known as sugars: Next to fats and proteins, this is one of the three major sources of energy obtained from food

GLYCEMIA: level of sugar in the blood.

INFUSION: way of preparing plants by boiling water and then steeping the plants in the water after removing the container from heat.

LIPIDS: also known as fats: Next to carbohydrates and proteins, this is one of the three sources of energy obtained from food.

MENOPAUSE: the period in women's lives where they stop having their periods for the rest of their lives.

METABOLISM: all the processes that transform substances and energy in the cells and body, leading to the synthesis or breaking down of biological substances.

NEUROTRANSMITTERS: chemical messengers which neurons produce for communication.

TRACE ELEMENTS: minerals found in trace amounts in the body.

OSTEOBLAST: bone cell found in cartilaginous tissue or cartilage which is developing into bone tissue.

OSTEOCLAST: large cells found along bones. Their role is to facilitate bone resorption.

OSTEOPOROSIS: disease characterized by bone weakness linked to decreased bone density, which increases the risk of bone fractures.

OVOCYTE: cell situated in the ovaries which can mature and develop into an ovum.

OVULATION: release of an ovum from the ovary. It can fuse with a spermatozoid, if one is present.

OVUM: female cell which can be fertilized and form an egg.

PHYTOESTROGEN: plant hormone with an effect similar to estrogens.

BLOOD PLATELETS: blood components which do not have a nucleus, and play an important role in blood clotting.

PROTEIN: next to fats and carbohydrates,

one of the three sources of energy obtained from food.

FREE RADICAL: molecule produced during oxidation, containing a free electron. This molecule looks for a neighboring molecule from which it "steals" an electron.

SERM: Selective Estrogen Receptor Modulator: drug with the particular ability to bind to cells with estrogen receptors. Once bound to them, the drug displays an activity that is different from that of estrogens, depending on the type of receptor.

SPERMATOGENESIS: the processes which lead to the formation of spermatozoids.

STEROIDS: group or hormonal substances with a common structure derived from sterols.

OXIDATIVE STRESS: aggression occurring inside the cells due to oxidative phenomena.

MOTHER TINCTURE: solution obtained by soaking plants in alcohol.

HRT (Hormone Replacement Therapy): treatment which entails taking hormones in order to replace the hormones which the body no longer produces or produces in insufficient quantities.

TRIGLYCERIDES: fats circulating in the blood. An increase in these fats is dependant on diet, particularly the intake of excess sugar and alcohol.

VITAMIN: substance essential for life, which the body cannot directly produce.

BIBLIOGRAPHY

Albertazzi P.: *The effect of dietary soy supplementation on hot flushes.* Obstetrics and Gynecology, 1998, 91: 6-10.

Anderson J.-W. : *Meta-analysis of the effects of soy protein intake on serum lipids.* The new England Journal of medicine, 1995, aug 3: 276-282.

Bezanger-Beauquesne L. : *Plantes médicinales des régions tempérées.* Maloine, Paris, 1990.

Chen C.: *Hormone replacement therapy in relation to breast cancer.* JAMA, 2002, 287: 734-741.

David H.-U. : *Vasomotor symptom relief by soy isoflavone extract tablets in postmenopausal women.* The Journal of the North American Menopause Society, 2000, 7 (4) : 236-242.

Drapier- Faure E.: *Effects of a standardized soy extract on hot flushes: a multicenter double blind, randomized, placebo-controlled study.* Menopause 2002, 9(5) : 329-334.

Fazzioli E. : *Les Jardins secrets de l'Empereur.* La Maison Rustique, Paris, 1990.

Fichaux B. : *La Nouvelle Cuisine familiale 150 menus, 300 recettes pour l'hiver.* GabriAndre, Saint-Jean-de-Valériscle, 1998.

Greenwood S. : *The role of isoflavones in menopausal health: consensus opinion of the north american menopause society.* The Journal of the North American Menopause Society, 2000, 7 (4), 215-229.

Hostettmann K. : *Tout savoir sur le pouvoir des plantes sources de médicaments.* Favre, Lausanne, 1997.

Joyeux H.: *Femmes, si vous saviez... (83 questions-réponses) Hormones-Ménopause- Ostéoporose.* François-Xavier de Guibert, Paris, 2001.

Lambert-Lagacé L.: *Ménopause, nutrition et santé.* Les Éditions de l'Homme, Montréal, 2000.

Lopes P., Trémollières F.: *Guide pratique de la ménopause.* MIMI Éditions, Masson, Paris, 2001.

Padrazzi P.: *L'Oligothérapie réactionnelle.* Similia, Paris, 1988.

Padrini F. et Lucheroni M.-T.: *Les Huiles essentielles pour retrouver la vitalité, le bien-être, la beauté.* De Vecchi, Paris, 1997.

Scambia G.: *Clinical effects of a standardized soy extract in postmenopausal women: a pilot study.* The Journal of the North American Menopause Society, 2000, vol.7, n° 2: 105-111.

Souccar T. et Curtay J.-P.: *Le Programme de longue vie.* Seuil, Paris, 1996.

Stoll B.-A.: *Eating to beat breast cancer : potential role for soy supplements.* Annal of oncology, 1997, 8: 223-225.

Taylor M.: *Alternatives to conventional hormone replacement therapy.* Comp Ther, 1997, 23(8) : 514-532.

Women's Health Initiative: Risks and benefits of estrogen plus progestin in healthy postmenopausal women. JAMA, 2002, 288 : 321-333.